SO-CBG-953

HEALTHCARE
CAREER STARTER

HEALTHCARE

career starter

2nd edition

Cheryl Hancock
with Brigit Dermott

New York

Library of Congress Cataloging-in-Publication Data:
Hancock, Cheryl
    Healthcare career starter / Cheryl Hancock with Brigit Dermott.—2nd ed.
        p. cm.
Previously published: Health care career starter.
        ISBN 1-57685-408-6
    1. Allied health personnel—Vocational guidance. I. Dermott, Brigit.
II. Hancock, Cheryl. Health care career starter. III. Title.
    R697.A4 H34 2002
    610.69—dc21

                                                    2002001275

Printed in the United States of America
9 8 7 6 5 4 3 2 1
Second Edition

ISBN 1-57685-408-6

For more information or to place an order, contact LearningExpress at:
    900 Broadway
    Suite 604
    New York, NY 10003

Or visit us at:
    www.learnatest.com

Contents

Contents

Introduction

Why Enter the Healthcare Field?

The healthcare industry is one of the fastest growing segments in the U.S. economy. Regardless of the strength of the economy, this field will continue to offer considerable employment opportunities. In fact, about 14 percent of all wage and salary jobs expected to be created by 2008 will be in health services. And out of the 30 occupations that are projected to grow the fastest, 12 are in healthcare. Currently, healthcare is one of the largest industries in the country—accounting for about 11.3 million jobs.

In addition, there are many other exciting reasons to pursue a career in healthcare. Because the healthcare industry has changed to become more cost conscious over the last decade, the healthcare job market has adjusted to meet the new climate. Employees are being given more responsibility earlier in their careers. This means that many of the new jobs in the healthcare field will be filled by employees with two years of training or less, and these employees will be more involved in direct patient care than in the past.

Along with increased cost consciousness, the healthcare market is changing as new medicine and technology alter the ways in which patients are treated. Such innovations as anesthesia that wears off quickly mean that the length of patients' hospital stays are reduced. In general, there is a movement away from hospital care to outpatient services and home care. This trend also contributes to the job opportunities for employees with two years of training or less. These trends do not mean that the quality of care is diminished. In fact, the move away from hospital care to home care can be a very positive trend for many patients, particularly the elderly.

Another important result of the increased demand for healthcare workers is improved earning potential. The average earnings for nonsupervisory workers in healthcare are higher than the average for all private industry. Hospital workers, who make up about 40 percent of all healthcare workers, earn substantially more on average. Even though there is movement away from hospital care, hospitals will continue to be the largest employers of healthcare workers. With the increased demand for healthcare workers in the years ahead, the earning potential will only get better.

In this book you will learn all about getting started in this exciting field. In Chapter 1, you will discover the hottest careers in the field that require a maximum of two years of training. The next chapter is devoted to helping you decide if a career in healthcare is right for you, and if so, to which particular job you are best suited. Chapter 3 gives you details about getting the training you need to pursue your new career, and Chapter 4 provides a wealth of information about financing your training.

The balance of the book will help you find your first job and then succeed in your new career. Chapter 5 offers important strategies for finding job opportunities and Chapter 6 will help you write a convincing cover letter and resume and make a great impression in an interview, so you will get hired in the job of your choice. In Chapter 7, you will learn how to succeed in your new career with special tips for meeting the challenges of healthcare work. Finally, in Chapter 8 you will find information about the most important trend in healthcare—gerontology.

This is a step-by-step guide to starting a career in healthcare from deciding on a field to getting training and from finding and winning a job to succeeding and getting ahead. You will also find a wealth of resources in the back of the book that will point you to organizations, websites, and books that can help you get your career started, achieve your training goals, and support you throughout your career.

There has never been a better time to enter the healthcare field. Even more than the job opportunities and earning potential, healthcare is a career that offers tremendous job satisfaction. It is a career devoted to helping others and it provides a vital service in the community. Now is also a time of great innovation in the field. Doctors and researchers are continually making discoveries and advancements that are improving the quality of care and overall life expectancy.

Read on to learn more about the important and exciting careers in the healthcare field.

HEALTHCARE
CAREER STARTER

CHAPTER one

THE HOTTEST HEALTHCARE CAREERS

THIS CHAPTER DESCRIBES the hottest entry-level healthcare careers. You will learn which jobs are expected to experience the most growth in the upcoming years. For each of these hot jobs, there is a detailed job description, and information about typical salary, advancement opportunities, hiring trends, and the skills needed for each job. You will also find a comprehensive list of the different areas of specialization in the healthcare field. And you will hear about the medical field from a real healthcare worker.

ACCORDING TO the United States Department of Labor, the healthcare industry is growing at an enormous rate. This means that now is an excellent time to consider a career in healthcare. People who pursue training in the following healthcare jobs are almost guaranteed to find employment in the years ahead: home health aide, nursing aide, physical therapy assistant, medical assistant, radiologic technician, medical records technician, surgical technician, and respiratory therapist.

There are two important factors contributing to the growing need for healthcare workers—the rise of managed care and the aging of the U.S. population. Under the managed care system, the healthcare industry looks for more efficient and cost-effective ways to provide care for patients. This means an increased role and need for aides and technicians who are trained to give basic care and assist doctors and nurses. A swiftly aging population also creates a more immediate need for aides and technicians who provide basic care but do not spend years in training like a nurse or a doctor.

All the jobs mentioned in the previous paragraph require some training, but in almost all cases you can become fully qualified in two years or less. This is one thing these jobs have in common. As you read on, you will discover that these jobs also have many important differences. Some are office jobs, others work directly with patients, and others still work with technical equipment. Reading these job descriptions—including salary and advancement opportunities—will help you understand the range of possibilities for someone starting a career in healthcare. To ensure accuracy and currency of the job descriptions, the information in the next sections is adapted from the most up-to-date *Occupational Outlook Handbook*, published by the U.S. Bureau of Labor Statistics.

HOME HEALTH AIDE

Job Description

Home health aides help people who require medical assistance to live in their own homes. Most often they work with elderly, disabled, and ill people. Home health aides provide health-related services, personal care, help around the house, and emotional support.

As part of their medical duties, home health aides:

▶ administer oral medications under physicians' orders or direction of a nurse and assist with medication routines
▶ check pulse, temperature, and respiration
▶ help with simple prescribed exercises, and give massages and alcohol rubs
▶ change nonsterile dressings
▶ use special equipment such as a hydraulic lift, or assist with braces and artificial limbs

Most home health aides also:

▶ do some housework such as cleaning, doing laundry, and changing the sheets
▶ help their clients with personal care such as bathing, dressing, and grooming
▶ plan meals (including special diets), shop for food, and cook

Companionship is an important part of a home health aide's job.

▶ They might accompany their clients when they travel outside their homes.
▶ They can also provide support for their clients' family members.
▶ They listen to their clients and keep them company.

Home health aides usually work through home care agencies. They work with a case manager—most often a registered nurse, a physical therapist, or a social worker—who supervises the patient's care. Home health aides also keep records about their clients' progress and condition.

Because home health aides work in other people's homes, their work environment and their daily routine can be quite varied. Depending on the needs of their clients, home health aides can work for one person for years or see as many as five different clients a day. For the most part, home health aides work alone and check in with their supervising agency. Clients can also range from depressed or angry to pleasant and cooperative. Work hours can also vary, and many home health aides work part-time.

Required Training

In some states, this occupation is open to individuals with no formal training; in other states some formal training is required. In addition to prior training, home health care agencies usually provide on-the-job training.

The federal government has required that home health aides whose employers receive reimbursement through the Medicare program pass a competency test. To pass the test, 75 hours of classroom and practical training supervised by a registered nurse is recommended. Training and testing programs may be offered by the employing agency. LearningExpress offers test preparation in book and online formats. Go to *www.LearnATest.com* to check these products out.

Home health aides can also obtain certification through the National Association for Home Care to show that their skills meet the industry standards. This certification is voluntary.

Hiring Trends

Home health and personal care aides held about 368,000 jobs in 1998, and the number is expected to increase by almost 75 percent by 2008. It is one of the fastest growing jobs in the United States. Most aides are employed by home healthcare agencies and visiting nurse associations. They are also employed by residential care facilities, hospitals, public health and welfare departments, community volunteer agencies, nursing and personal care facilities, and temporary help firms.

Earning Potential

Most home health aides are paid an hourly wage and they often do not receive benefits. In 2000, a typical hourly wage was between $7 and $9 an hour.

Annual earnings in the following cities in 2000 for the lower half, the median, and the top half of earners were:

	Lower Half	Median	Top Half
Charlotte, NC	$15,211	$18,819	$23,260
El Paso, TX	$13,987	$17,305	$21,388
Jacksonville, FL	$14,514	$17,957	$22,194
Los Angeles, CA	$17,302	$21,406	$26,457
Milwaukee, WI	$16,203	$20,046	$24,775
New York, NY	$18,302	$22,146	$26,675
San Francisco, CA	$18,077	$22,364	$27,641

Who Makes a Good Home Health Aide?

A successful home health aide must enjoy helping people and be willing to work hard. It can be demanding work and a home healthcare aide does not have the immediate support of coworkers. An ideal home health aide is:

▶ responsible and emotionally stable
▶ compassionate and upbeat
▶ tactful, honest, and discreet
▶ in good health and reasonably strong

Career Outlook

Advancement for home health aides is limited. As they gain experience, home health aides can expect salary increases, but the earning potential in this career remains fairly low. But because the required training is minimal and can sometimes be obtained on the job, this job can be a great choice for someone who is interested in healthcare but is not ready to commit to more advanced training. The experience gained as a home health aide will be helpful when applying to programs for more advanced careers and when looking for work in another healthcare field.

NURSING AIDE OR NURSING ASSISTANT

Job Description

Nursing aides help care for people confined to hospitals, or nursing and residential care facilities. Psychiatric aides, whose duties are very similar to nursing aides, help care for the mentally ill in mental health facilities. Nursing aides are also known as nursing assistants, geriatric aides, unlicensed assistive personnel, or hospital attendants.

They perform routine tasks under the supervision of nursing and medical staff. They:

▶ answer patients' call bells and deliver messages
▶ serve meals and help patients eat
▶ dress and bathe patients, and make beds

Aides may also:

▶ take temperatures, pulse, respiration, and blood pressure
▶ help patients get in and out of bed and walk
▶ provide skin care to patients
▶ escort patients to operating and examining rooms
▶ keep patients' rooms neat
▶ set up equipment, and store and move supplies

Nursing aides also observe patients' physical, mental, and emotional conditions and report any change to the nursing or medical staff.

A nursing aide can work either full or part time. Because patients need 24-hour care, aides often work evenings, nights, weekends, and holidays. Nursing aides are often on their feet and can be required to do some heavy lifting. Although they often have unpleasant duties, such as emptying bedpans and caring for irritable patients, many aides find helping others very satisfying. Some aides, especially those who work in nursing homes, are their patients' primary caregivers.

Required Training

In many cases, no formal training is required. It is not always necessary to have a high school diploma or previous work experience. Hospitals, however, may require prior experience as a nursing aide or home health aide, and some states require psychiatric aides to complete a formal training program. Nursing homes often provide training for new employees who may be required to pass a competency test within four months of being hired.

Some facilities other than nursing homes provide classroom instruction for newly hired aides, while others rely exclusively on informal on-the-job instruction from a licensed nurse or an experienced aide. Such training may last several days to a few months. From time to time, aides may also attend lectures, workshops, and in-service training.

Hiring Trends

Nursing aides held about 1.4 million jobs in 2000, and that number is expected to increase by almost 25 percent by 2008. About one-half of all nursing aides work in nursing homes, and about one-fourth work in hospitals. Others work in residential care facilities or in private households.

Earning Potential

Hourly wages for nursing aides in 1998 on average ranged from $7 to $10 an hour. Paid holidays and sick leave, hospital and medical benefits, extra pay for late-shift work, and pension plans are available to many hospital and some nursing home employees. Nursing aides can often earn additional wages for overtime work. In 2000, the annual salaries of nursing aides in the United States ranged from $13,480 to $26,390, with the average salary around $18,500. Annual earnings for certified physical therapy assistants in the following cities in 2000 for the lower half, the median, and the top half of earners were:

	Lower Half	Median	Top Half
Denver, CO	$15,667	$21,760	$29,889
Indianapolis, IN	$15,012	$20,850	$29,607
Sacramento, CA	$14,529	$20,180	$28,655
Tucson, AZ	$13.284	$18,450	$26,199
Washington, DC	$15,250	$21,180	$30,075

Who Makes a Good Nursing Aide?

Nursing aides work directly with patients and also work closely with other medical personnel, including doctors and nurses. Because their primary responsibility is to provide patient care, aides should be:

- ▶ tactful and patient
- ▶ compassionate and emotionally stable
- ▶ reliable and a team player
- ▶ dedicated to helping people
- ▶ have good communication skills
- ▶ willing to perform repetitive, routine tasks

Career Outlook

The opportunities for advancement occupations open to nursing aides are limited. However, some employers and unions help nursing aides obtain the education they need to advance into other healthcare careers. Working as a nursing aide can help you decide whether you want to pursue a more advanced career in the healthcare field, and the experience will help you when applying for a program and future employment.

PHYSICAL THERAPY ASSISTANT AND AIDE

Job Description

Physical therapist assistants and aides help physical therapists provide treatments that improve mobility, relieve pain, and prevent or limit permanent disability in patients suffering from injuries or disease. Patients include accident victims and people with various conditions, such as lower back pain, arthritis, muscular and skeletal injuries, and cerebral palsy.

Physical therapist assistants perform a variety of tasks under the direction of therapists. They:

▶ help patients with therapeutic exercises
▶ give massages and electrical stimulation to ease muscle pain
▶ give paraffin baths
▶ apply hot and cold packs
▶ use traction and ultrasound

They also record the patient's responses to treatment and report to the physical therapist the outcome of each treatment.

Physical therapist aides help make therapy sessions productive. They are usually responsible for:

▶ keeping the treatment area clean and organized
▶ preparing for each patient's therapy
▶ assisting patients in moving to or from a treatment area
▶ ordering supplies
▶ answering the phone
▶ filling out insurance forms and other paperwork

Because they are not licensed, aides perform a more limited range of tasks than physical therapist assistants do. A physical therapist assistant might also fill the role of an aide at some smaller clinics.

Recommended Training

Physical therapist aides are usually required to have a high school diploma and then receive training on the job. Physical therapist assistants typically have earned an associate's degree from a two-year accredited physical therapist assistant program. Additional requirements include certification in CPR and other first aid and a minimum number of hours of clinical experience.

Hiring Trends

Physical therapist assistants and aides held 82,000 jobs in 1998 and almost 45 percent growth is expected through 2008. Over two-thirds of all assistants and aides work in hospitals or offices of physical therapists. Others work in nursing and personal care facilities, outpatient rehabilitation centers, offices and clinics of physicians, and home health agencies.

Earnings

Annual earnings of physical therapist assistants and aides ranged from $13,760 to more than $39,730 in 1998, and the median annual salary was about $20,000. Physical therapy assistants can typically expect to earn more than aides. Annual earnings for certified physical therapy assistants in the following cities in 2000 for the lower half, the median, and the top half of earners were:

	Lower Half	Median	Top Half
Detroit, MI	$32,707	$37,702	$43,550
Jacksonville, FL	$27,911	$32,174	$37,164
Los Angeles, CA	$33,273	$38,354	$44,304
Philadelphia, PA	$31,546	$36,363	$42,003
San Antonio, TX	$27,762	$32,002	$36,966
San Diego, CA	$31,218	$35,985	$41,567

Who Makes a Good Physical Therapy Assistant or Aide?

One important characteristic of physical therapist assistants and aides is fitness. They need to have a moderate degree of strength due to the physical exertion required in assisting patients with their treatment. Assistants and aides may need to help lift patients, and kneeling, stooping, and standing for long periods are all part of the job.

Someone interested in becoming a physical therapy assistant should also have good academic skills, as admission to training programs can be quite competitive.

Like all healthcare workers, both assistants and aides should be interested in helping people, and have patience and compassion. Because physical therapy involves encouraging patients to complete exercises to aid in their recovery, physical therapy assistants and aides should be good motivators with upbeat personalities. Physical therapy aides should also have good attention to detail because it is often their job to keep the office running smoothly.

Career Outlook

Within the physical therapy profession, advancement comes with training. Aides become assistants by becoming certified, and assistants become therapists by completing an advanced course of study. Because this is a high-growth field, prospects for newly certified physical therapy assistants will be very good in the years ahead.

MEDICAL ASSISTANT

Job Description

Medical assistants perform the administrative and clinical tasks that keep the offices and clinics of physicians, podiatrists, chiropractors, optometrists, and other medical specialists running smoothly. The duties of medical assistants vary depending on office location, size, and specialty. In small practices, a medical assistant might handle both administrative and clinical tasks. In a larger practice, medical assistants tend to specialize in either administrative or clinical duties. Administrative duties of medical assistants include:

- ▶ answering the telephone, greeting patients, and scheduling appointments
- ▶ keeping patients' medical records, filling out insurance forms, handling correspondence, billing, and bookkeeping
- ▶ arranging for hospital admission and laboratory services

Clinical duties vary according to state law and can include a wide variety of tasks such as:

▶ taking medical histories and recording temperature, blood pressure, and pulse

▶ preparing patients for examination, explaining treatment procedures to patients, and assisting the physician during the examination

▶ collecting and preparing laboratory specimens, and performing basic laboratory and diagnostic tests including drawing blood, preparing patients for X rays, and taking electrocardiograms

▶ removing sutures and changing dressings

▶ instructing patients about medication and special diets and preparing and administering medications as directed by a physician

▶ authorizing drug refills as directed and calling in prescriptions to a pharmacy

▶ arranging, purchasing, and maintaining examining room instruments and equipment, disposing of contaminated supplies, and sterilizing medical instruments

Recommended Training

Most employers prefer to hire graduates of formal programs in medical assisting. These programs are offered in vocational–technical high schools, postsecondary vocational schools, community and junior colleges, and in colleges and universities. Programs last either one year, resulting in a certificate or diploma, or two years, resulting in an associate degree. Accredited programs include an internship that provides practical experience in physicians' offices, hospitals, or other healthcare facilities.

Formal training is an important advantage and is becoming almost a necessity. Employers prefer to hire experienced workers or certified applicants who have passed a national examination showing that they meet industry standards of competence. However, some medical assistants are trained on the job. Applicants without formal training usually need a high school diploma, and volunteer experience in the healthcare field is also helpful.

Hiring Trends

The good news is that medical assisting is expected to be one of the 10 fastest growing occupations through the year 2008. Medical assistants held about 252,000 jobs in 1998, and that number is expected to increase by almost 60 percent. About 65 percent of medical assistants work in physicians' offices, and 15 percent work in offices of other health practitioners such as chiropractors, optometrists, and podiatrists. The remaining 20 percent work in hospitals, nursing homes, and other healthcare facilities. Job prospects will be best for medical assistants with formal training or experience, particularly those with certification.

Earning Potential

Medical assistants' salaries depend on their level of experience, their skill level, and where they work. The median salary for a medical assistant in 1998 was $20,680, and salaries ranged from just over $14,000 to almost $29,000. Medical assistants working for physicians or in hospitals tend to earn slightly more than those who work for other healthcare practitioners.

Annual earnings for certified physical therapy assistants in the following cities in 2000 for the lower half, the median, and the top half of earners were:

	Lower Half	Median	Top Half
Birmingham, AL	$16,118	$22,080	$31,574
Boston, MA	$20,834	$28,540	$40,812
Chicago, IL	$20,162	$27,620	$39,496
Miami, FL	$16,563	$22,690	$32,446
Milwaukee, WI	$18,622	$25,510	$36,479
Seattle, WA	$19,366	$26,530	$37,937

Who Makes a Good Medical Assistant?

Medical assistants work directly with patients and conduct business for their offices so they must be:

▶ neat and courteous
▶ able to put patients at ease and explain physicians' instructions
▶ trustworthy and able to keep medical information confidential
▶ capable of handling several responsibilities at once
▶ clinical duties require a reasonable level of manual dexterity, and good eyesight.

Career Outlook

Medical assistants may be able to advance to office manager. A manager supervises the medical assistants, has a higher level of responsibility, and, as a result, can expect to earn a higher salary. Medical assistants are qualified to fill a wide variety of administrative support jobs, and they can teach medical assisting. With some additional education, medical assistants can also enter other health occupations such as nursing and medical technology.

RADIOLOGIC TECHNOLOGIST

Job Description

Radiologic technologists use special equipment to take diagnostic images of patients that doctors use to learn about patients' condition. X rays, sono-grams, and magnetic resonance imaging (MRI), are the most common diag-nostic imaging techniques. The two main types of radiographic technologists are radiographers and sonographers.

Radiographers take X rays, or radiographs. They:

▶ explain the procedure, remove clothing such as jewelry through which X rays cannot pass, and position the patient

▶ protect patients from unnecessary radiation exposure with devices such as lead shields, or by limiting the size of the X ray beam

▶ position the equipment at the correct angle and height and set controls on the machine to produce radiographs of the appropriate density, detail, and contrast

▶ place the X ray film under the part of the patient's body to be examined, make the exposure, and then remove the film and develop it.

Experienced radiographers may perform more complicated imaging tests, such as fluoroscopies. In this procedure, radiographers prepare a solution of contrast medium for the patient to drink. This fluid shows up on an X ray and allows the radiologist, a physician who interprets radiographs, to see soft tissues in the body. Some radiographers, called CT technologists, operate computerized tomography scanners to produce cross sectional views of patients. Others operate machines that use giant magnets and radio waves rather than radiation to create an image. They are called magnetic resonance imaging (MRI) technologists.

Sonographers, also known as ultrasonographers, operate equipment that uses high frequency sound waves to create an image from the reflected echoes. Unlike an X ray, which is a still picture, a sonogram is viewed "live" on a screen and may be recorded on videotape or photographed for interpretation and diagnosis by physicians. Sonographers:

▶ explain the procedure and record the patient's medical history

▶ select appropriate equipment settings and use various patient positions as necessary

▶ view the screen as the scan takes place and decide which images to include in a videotape or still picture

▶ judge if the images are satisfactory for diagnostic purposes

Sonographers may specialize in neurosonography (the brain), vascular (blood flows), echocardiography (the heart), abdominal (the liver, kidneys, spleen, and pancreas), obstetrics/gynecology (the female reproductive system), or ophthalmology (the eye).

In addition to preparing patients and operating equipment, radiologic technologists:

▶ keep patient records and adjust and maintain equipment
▶ prepare work schedules
▶ evaluate equipment purchases

Most full-time radiologic technologists work about 40 hours a week, but they may have evening, weekend, or on-call hours.

Recommended Training

Hospitals, which employ most radiologic technologists, prefer to hire people with formal training. Programs in radiography and diagnostic medical sonography (ultrasound) range in length from one to four years and lead to a certificate, associate's degree, or bachelor's degree. Two-year associate's degree programs are most common.

Experienced radiographers or individuals from other health occupations who want to change fields or specialize in sonography can become certified in one year. A bachelor's or master's degree in one of the radiologic technologies is desirable for supervisory, administrative, or teaching positions.

To enter a radiography program you must have, at a minimum, a high school diploma or the equivalent. For training programs in diagnostic medical sonography, applicants with a background in science or experience in one of the health professions generally are preferred. Some programs consider applicants with liberal arts backgrounds, however, as well as high school graduates with courses in math and science.

In 1999, 35 states and Puerto Rico required radiologic technologists to be licensed. Sonographers are not required to be licensed. Voluntary registration is offered by the American Registry of Radiologic Technologists (ARRT) in radiography. The American Registry of Diagnostic Medical Sonographers (ARDMS) certifies the competence of sonographers. To be eligible for registration, technologists generally must graduate from an accredited program and pass an examination. Many employers prefer to hire registered radiographers and sonographers.

Radiographers must complete 24 hours of continuing education every other year and sonographers must complete 30 hours of continuing education every three years.

Hiring Trends

Radiologic technologists held about 162,000 jobs in 1998; that number is expected to increase by almost 20 percent by 2008. The majority of technologists were employed as radiographers. More than 50 percent of technologists work in hospitals and the rest work in physicians' offices and clinics, including diagnostic imaging centers.

Sonographers should experience somewhat better job opportunities than radiographers because ultrasound is becoming an increasingly attractive alternative to radiologic procedures. Radiologic technologists who are educated and have credentials in more than one type of imaging technology will have better employment opportunities.

Earning Potential

Radiologic technologists earned an average of about $33,000 in 1998. Annual earnings for radiologic technologist in the following cities in 2000 for the lower half, the median, and the top half of earners were:

	Lower Half	Median	Top Half
Detroit, MI	$32,151	$36,002	$42,228
Houston, TX	$30,453	$34,100	$39,997
Indianapolis, IN	$29,135	$32,624	$38,267
Los Angeles, CA	$32,708	$36,625	$42,959
New York, NY	$33,820	$37,871	$44,420
San Francisco, CA	$34,172	$38,264	$44,882

Who Makes a Good Radiologic Technologist?

Radiologic technologists must follow physicians' orders precisely and conform to regulations concerning use of radiation to protect themselves, their patients, and coworkers from unnecessary exposure. An ideal radiologic technologist is:

▶ patient and capable of carefully explaining procedures
▶ good with math and science
▶ precise, with careful attention to detail

Career Outlook

There is great potential for growth in the field of radiologic technology. With experience and additional training, technologists may become specialists, performing CT scanning, angiography, and magnetic resonance imaging. Experienced technologists may also be promoted to supervisor or chief radiologic technologist, and, ultimately, department administrator or director. Sometimes additional courses or a master's degree in business or health administration may be necessary to advance to the level of director. Some technologists progress by becoming instructors or directors in radiologic technology programs; others take jobs as sales representatives or instructors with equipment manufacturers.

MEDICAL RECORDS TECHNICIAN

Job Description

Medical records are an essential part of treating patients. A medical record includes information about a patient's medical history, observations about the patient's current condition, and suggestions and notes for a course of treatment. These records help physicians and other medical personnel to understand a patient's case and make assessments. Medical records technicians organize and evaluate these records for completeness and accuracy.

Medical record technicians are also called health information technicians. They:

▶ make sure a patient's initial medical chart is complete, ensure all forms are complete and properly identified and signed, and enter all necessary information into a computer

▶ assign a code to each diagnosis and procedure

▶ use a software program to assign the patient to one of several hundred diagnosis-related groups, or DRG's, which determine insurance reimbursement

▶ use computer programs to tabulate and analyze data for various uses such as improving patient care, controlling costs, or responding to surveys

Medical record technicians usually work a 40-hour week. Their hours may be more regular than healthcare workers involved in direct patient care, but hospital medical records departments are open almost all the time. These technicians may work day, evening, and night shifts.

Recommended Training

An associate degree from a community or junior college is usually required for medical records technicians. Hospitals sometimes advance promising health information clerks to jobs as health information technicians, although this practice may be less common in the future.

In addition to an associate degree, most employers prefer applicants to have accreditation. In order to become an Accredited Record Technician (ART), applicants must graduate from an accredited two-year program and then pass a written test. Technicians who specialize in coding may also obtain voluntary certification.

Hiring Trends

Medical records technician is projected to be one of the 20 fastest-growing occupations through 2008. There were about 92,000 medical records technicians in 1998. About two of every five of these worked in hospitals. Most others worked in nursing homes, medical group practices, clinics, and home health agencies. Insurance firms and public health departments also employ a small number of medical records technicians to tabulate and analyze health information.

Earning Potential

Medical records technicians earned between about $17,000 and $31,000 a year in 1998. Annual earnings for medical records technicians in the following cities in 2000 for the lower half, the median, and the top half of earners were:

	Lower Half	Median	Top Half
Austin, TX	$22,735	$26,647	$31,253
Boston, MA	$25,901	$30,358	$35,605
Charlotte, NC	$23,378	$27,401	$32,137
Columbus, OH	$24,901	$29,186	$34,231
Milwaukee, WI	$24,901	$29,186	$34,231
Seattle, WA	$25,758	$30,191	$34,090

Who Makes a Good Medical Records Technician?

Unlike many other jobs in the medical field, a medical records technician does not need to have the personal skills necessary to work well with patients. The most important trait for a medical records technician is the ability to pay close attention to detail. Accuracy is essential, so technicians must be organized and meticulous about their work. Medical records technicians often use computers to organize data. A person who is interested in working with computers and with statistics will be well suited to medical records.

Career Outlook

Experienced medical records technicians usually advance in one of two ways—by specializing or managing. Many senior medical records technicians specialize in coding, particularly Medicare coding, or in tumor registry, which aids cancer researchers in gathering data about disease and treatment.

In large medical records departments, experienced technicians may advance to section supervisor, and oversee the work of other coders. Senior technicians with Accredited Record Technicians (ART) credentials may become director or assistant director of a health information department in a small facility. However, in larger institutions, the director must have a bachelor's degree.

SURGICAL TECHNOLOGIST

Job Description

Surgical technologists, who are also called surgical or operating room technicians, assist during operations under the supervision of surgeons, registered nurses, or other surgical personnel. Before an operation, surgical technologists:

▶ help set up the operating room with surgical instruments and equipment, sterile linens, and sterile solutions
▶ sssemble, adjust, and check nonsterile equipment to ensure it is working properly
▶ prepare patients for surgery by washing, shaving, and disinfecting incision sites
▶ transport patients to the operating room, help position them on the operating table, and cover them with sterile surgical drapes
▶ observe patients' vital signs, check charts, and help the surgical team scrub and put on gloves, gowns, and masks

During surgery, technologists:

▶ pass instruments and other sterile supplies to surgeons and surgeon assistants
▶ may hold retractors, cut sutures, and help count sponges, needles, supplies, and instruments
▶ help prepare, care for, and dispose of specimens taken for laboratory analysis and may help apply dressings
▶ some operate sterilizers, lights, or suction machines, and help operate diagnostic equipment
▶ may also maintain supplies of fluids, such as plasma and blood

After an operation, surgical technologists may help transfer patients to the recovery room and clean and restock the operating room.

Recommended Training

Surgical technologists are required to graduate from a formal training program lasting from nine to 24 months. These training programs are offered by community and junior colleges, vocational schools, universities, hospitals, and the military. High school graduation is generally required for admission. Graduates earn a certificate, diploma, or associate degree. Students who are already licensed practical nurses or military personnel with appropriate training may qualify for shorter training programs.

Training programs provide a balance of classroom instruction—including anatomy, physiology, microbiology, pharmacology, professional ethics, and medical terminology—and supervised clinical experience. Students learn about the care and safety of patients during surgery, aseptic techniques, and surgical procedures. They are also instructed in procedures such as sterilizing instruments; preventing and controlling infection; and handling special drugs, solutions, supplies, and equipment.

Technologists who graduate from a formal program and pass a national certification examination can obtain professional certification from the Liaison Council on Certification for the Surgical Technologist. They may then use the designation Certified Surgical Technologist, or CST. Continuing education or reexamination is required to maintain certification, which must be renewed every six years. Most employers prefer to hire certified technologists.

Hiring Trends

Surgical technologists held about 54,000 jobs in 1998 and this number is expected to increase by over 40 percent by 2008. Most technologists are employed by hospitals, mainly in operating and delivery rooms. Others are employed in clinics and surgical centers, and in the offices of physicians and dentists who perform outpatient surgery.

Earning Potential

In 1998, surgical technologists earned between about $19,000 and $35,000 a year with an average annual income of about $25,000.

Annual earnings surgical technologists in the following cities in 2000 for the lower half, the median, and the top half of earners were:

	Lower Half	Median	Top Half
Detroit, MI	$26,821	$31,303	$35,380
Indianapolis, IN	$24,305	$28,367	$32,061
Jacksonville, FL	$22,306	$26,145	$30,664
Philadelphia, PA	$25,868	$30,192	$34,123
San Francisco, CA	$28,506	$33,271	$37,603
San Jose, CA	$28,286	$33,014	$37,313

Who Makes a Good Surgical Technologist?

Surgical technologists must have good manual dexterity so they can handle instruments quickly. They also must be conscientious, orderly, and emotionally stable because the operating room is a very demanding work environment. A good surgical technologist will also be able to respond quickly as situations arise and thoroughly understand procedures so they can anticipate a surgeon's needs. A candidate for a career as a surgical technologist should have an interest in science and strong academic skills. A person who is quick-witted, capable, and responds well to stress will have a good future in this field.

Career Outlook

Technologists advance by specializing in a particular area of surgery, such as neurosurgery or open heart surgery. With additional training, some technologists advance to first assistants, who help with retracting, sponging, suturing, cauterizing bleeders, and closing and treating wounds. Some surgical technologists manage central supply departments in hospitals, or take positions with insurance companies, sterile supply services, and operating equipment firms.

RESPIRATORY THERAPIST

Job Description

Respiratory therapists evaluate, treat, and care for patients with breathing disorders. They treat all types of patients, from premature infants whose lungs are not fully developed to elderly people whose lungs are diseased.

Often working closely with the supervision of a physician, they:

▶ evaluate patients by testing lung capacity and analyzing oxygen and carbon dioxide concentration
▶ test the patient's blood (and in many cases draw the blood for the test) for potential of hydrogen (pH), which indicates the level of acidity or alkalinity
▶ increase a patient's concentration of oxygen using an oxygen mask or nasal cannula
▶ connect patients who cannot breathe on their own to ventilators that deliver pressurized oxygen into the lungs

▶ regularly check on patients and equipment and make adjustments if the patient is having difficulty

In home care, respiratory therapists teach patients and their families to use ventilators and other life support systems. Additionally, they visit several times a month to inspect and clean equipment and ensure its proper use. They may make emergency visits if equipment problems arise. Therapists also keep records of materials used and charges to patients.

Respiratory therapists also perform chest physiotherapy on patients to remove mucus from their lungs and make it easier for them to breathe. Chest physiotherapy helps patients suffering from lung diseases, such as cystic fibrosis, that cause mucus to collect in the lungs. In this procedure, therapists place patients in positions to help drain mucus, thump and vibrate patients' rib cages, and instruct them to cough.

Recently, respiratory therapists' role has expanded. They may also perform cardiopulmonary (heart and lung) procedures like electrocardiograms and stress testing.

Respiratory therapists generally work between 35 and 40 hours a week. Because hospitals operate around the clock, therapists may work evenings, nights, or weekends.

Recommended Training

Formal training is necessary to enter this field. Some programs prepare graduates for jobs as registered respiratory therapists (RRT). These programs generally last two years and lead to an associate degree, although some are four-year, bachelor degree programs. Other, shorter programs lead to jobs as certified respiratory therapists (CRT). These programs generally last one year. In addition, many therapists receive on-the-job training, allowing them to administer electrocardiograms and stress tests, as well as draw blood samples from patients. In order to become an RRT and CRT, candidates must graduate from an accredited program and pass a national exam.

Most employers require applicants for entry-level or generalist positions to hold the CRT or be eligible to take the certification examination. Supervisory positions and those in intensive care specialties usually require the RRT (or RRT eligibility).

Hiring Trends

Respiratory therapists held about 86,000 jobs in 1998. Almost 90 percent of these workers were employed by hospitals. The remaining 10 percent worked for home health agencies, respiratory therapy clinics, and nursing homes. Because of the growing elderly population the number of jobs in this field is expected to increase by 43 percent by 2008.

Opportunities are expected to be highly favorable for respiratory therapists with cardiopulmonary care skills and experience working with infants.

Earning Potential

Respiratory therapists earned from almost $26,000 to over $46,000 a year in 1998. The median annual earning were $34,830 in 1998.

Annual earnings respiratory therapists in the following cities in 2000 for the lower half, the median, and the top half of earners were:

	Lower Half	Median	Top Half
Detroit, MI	$33,634	$40,914	$50,783
Indianapolis, IN	$30,479	$37,076	$46,019
Jacksonville, FL	$30,479	$37,076	$46,019
Los Angeles, CA	$34,217	$41,622	$51,661
New York, NY	$35,264	$42,896	$53,243
Phoenix, AZ	$30,081	$36,592	$45,418

Who Makes a Good Respiratory Therapist?

A respiratory therapist works directly with patients, so he or she must be sensitive and caring. A person who enjoys working with the elderly or newborn infants would be especially good in this field. Respiratory care also requires workers to pay attention to detail, follow instructions, and work well as part of a team. In addition, respiratory workers operate complicated respiratory therapy equipment and they need mechanical ability and manual dexterity to do their work well. Strong math and science skills are also a great benefit to a respiratory therapist.

An ideal respiratory therapist shows a balance of sensitivity and caring with a strong sense of detail and technical ability.

Career Outlook

Respiratory therapists advance by moving from care of general to critical patients who have significant problems in other organ systems, such as the heart or kidneys. Respiratory therapists, especially those with four-year degrees, may also advance to supervisory or managerial positions in a respiratory therapy department. Respiratory therapists in home care and equipment rental firms may advance by becoming branch managers.

OTHER HEALTHCARE CAREERS

The careers outlined above are among the most promising career choices in healthcare, but they are only a very limited selection of the many careers that you can pursue in this field. The range of jobs is tremendous. The jobs listed next will give you some idea of the scope of the field, but even this list does not include every job that can be found in healthcare. These jobs represent both ends of the training spectrum—from short training programs to advanced degrees. In many cases you can be an assistant or aide in the specialties listed below. For example, instead of being a physical therapy aide, you could be an art or dance therapy aide if you have an arts background.

- ▶ Art therapists are trained in the fine arts and the behavioral sciences to develop rehabilitation programs that use art materials and techniques (such as painting, sculpting with clay, and making crafts).
- ▶ Audiologists test, diagnose, and treat people who have hearing and related problems.

- ▶ Biochemists study and research the chemical composition of living things, focusing on processes such as metabolism, reproduction, growth, and heredity.

- ▶ Biomedical engineers use engineering skills and concepts to invent or improve devices, instruments, and substances (for example, pacemakers, ultrasound, and artificial limbs) used in treating medical problems.

- ▶ Blood bank technologists are medical technologists who specialize in the skills and knowledge needed to maintain a blood bank, such as drawing, classifying, testing, analyzing, and storing blood.

- ▶ Cardiopulmonary technologists conduct tests and evaluations related to the diagnosis and treatment of heart (cardiac) and lung (pulmonary) diseases and disorders.

- ▶ Cardiovascular technicians assist physicians and other medical personnel in diagnosing and treating medical problems related to the body's heart (cardiac) and blood vessel (peripheral vascular) systems.

- ▶ Chiropractors diagnose and treat medical problems related to the body's muscular, nervous, and skeletal systems, especially the spine.

- ▶ Dance therapists are trained in dance/movement, psychology, and physiology to treat and rehabilitate patients with emotional or physical disorders, or developmental disabilities.

- ▶ Dental hygienists perform preventive dental procedures, including cleaning teeth, and instruct patients on oral hygiene practices to prevent tooth and gum abnormalities or disease.

- ▶ Dentists diagnose, prevent, and treat problems of the teeth and tissues of the mouth.

- ▶ Dietitians plan nutrition programs and supervise meal preparation and service, often for large institutions such as hospitals, schools, nursing homes, and prisons.

- ▶ EEG technologists conduct tests using EEG (electroencephalograph) equipment, which records electrical impulses in the brain, to assist neurologists (physicians who study the brain) in treating patients with neural disorders such as brain tumors, strokes, and Alzheimer's disease.

- ▶ EKG technicians are cardiovascular technicians who perform EKG (electrocardiogram) testing to record and monitor electrical impulses transmitted by the heart.

▶ Genetic counselors advise patients, often prospective parents, on matters related to hereditary diseases and disorders such as Down Syndrome, muscular dystrophy, and prenatal spinal or organ malformations.

▶ Licensed practical nurses provide basic nursing care (both medical and nonmedical) to sick, injured, convalescing, and handicapped patients under the direction of physicians and registered nurses.

▶ Medical illustrators use artistic skills and medical and anatomical knowledge to create drawings, diagrams, models, and other graphic aids for use in medical research, publications, consultations, exhibits, teaching, and various communications media.

▶ Optometrists diagnose and treat vision problems, prescribing and fitting eyeglasses and contact lenses, and may provide basic care for eye disorders such as cataracts and glaucoma (unlike ophthalmologists, however, who are physicians specializing in the treatment of eye diseases and injuries).

▶ Orthotists design, build, and fit devices to support weak body parts or correct physical defects, such as limb or spinal cord disorders stemming from cerebral palsy, polio, or stroke.

▶ Pharmacists dispense drugs prescribed by physicians and other medical practitioners, advise patients about medications, and consult with physicians about the selection, dosages, and effects of medications.

▶ Physical therapists rehabilitate people who suffer from physical disabilities caused by accidents or disease, using massage, water instruction, machine movement, or other methods.

▶ Podiatrists are doctors who diagnose and treat disorders, diseases, and injuries of the foot and lower leg.

▶ Prosthetists design, build, and fit artificial limbs (prostheses) for patients who have lost part or all of their own limbs due to accident, illness, or a congenital condition.

▶ Psychologists study human behavior and mental processes to understand, explain, and change people's behavior, often within an area of specialty such as clinical, developmental, organizational, or research psychology.

▶ Recreation therapists use games, sports, exercises, arts and crafts, and other recreational activities to treat patients with emotional, physical, or mental disorders and help them develop effective social and interpersonal skills.

▶ Registered nurses provide direct and indirect patient care, including assessing, planning, implementing, and evaluating care in areas ranging from pediatrics to geriatrics.

▶ Respiratory therapists evaluate, treat, and care for patients with breathing disorders such as asthma and emphysema and provide emergency care for heart failure, stroke, drowning, or shock victims.

▶ Surgeons work in the operating rooms of hospitals performing surgery on patients. Many surgeons specialize in a particular area of the body.

Now that you have an idea of the types of careers that you can pursue in healthcare, you might be wondering how to decide which career is right for you. The jobs we've covered are quite different in terms of how much training is required, earning potential, opportunity for advancement, and the personal qualities that make a person successful in each job. In order to find the best match with your needs, aspirations, and personality, you need to make an honest assessment of who you are, where you are at this point in your life, and where you would like to be. The next chapter is designed to help you make this assessment and, once you have determined which job is right for you, to help you find out more about the career you have chosen.

THE INSIDE TRACK

Who: Michael Adams
What: Respiratory Technician
Where: Chicago, Illinois

INSIDER'S STORY

I work in an urgent care outpatient clinic in downtown Chicago. Many of the patients that come in for respiratory therapy are kids with acute asthma. Asthma patients get priority treatment because if they can't breathe, they can lose consciousness. So, when I'm on duty, I am permanently on call. If I'm on a break, I must return immediately to the admissions area. My speed in answering my page can have serious consequences.

My other main category of patients are elderly and they often suffer from emphysema. Again, timely therapy is what they are here for, and it's my duty to get them breathing comfortably. My job is pretty demanding and you could say that I'm under pressure. We all are. In a way, that urgency feeds into our systems and we actually get energized on the job, knowing that it's all about saving lives.

I have certification as a respiratory technician, which I received after a one-year program. My goal is to go back to school full time and get advanced certification in respiratory therapy and take courses in pediatric care. I really like working with the kids that come in, and it's great to know that you helped them breathe. Also, I think that there's not enough awareness in the community about asthma and how to control symptoms. If parents understood the disease better and had better access to preventative medicines, then it's likely that their kids wouldn't be coming in here so frequently in distress. I have read about programs in other cities where a staff of specialists go around to the public schools and talk to the students about asthma. I would like to be involved in a program like this, and I'm starting to talk to some of the doctors here about getting something started in Chicago.

My advice for someone getting into this specialty is to pay attention in class and practice. Working with the equipment seems easy enough, but we don't just push a button and give oxygen to patients. Accuracy is important and you have to be good at math. Also, many of the kids and adults are in full distress about not being able to breathe and panic. Remaining calm in an emergency situation is really important. If you start rushing and fumbling with equipment, even if you know everything will be OK, a patient can get even more anxious. Being able to stay cool under pressure means that you might have what it takes to be a respiratory technician.

CHAPTER two

FINDING THE CAREER THAT'S RIGHT FOR YOU

THE HEALTHCARE FIELD is an explosive arena for job growth. But the field is very diverse. In this chapter you will discover which job is right for you, learn who hires entry-level healthcare workers, and find important tips on researching your career and the available training. Before you take the next step—getting the necessary training—you need to learn more about yourself and the career you want to pursue. This chapter will help you accomplish of these tasks.

AS YOU discovered in Chapter 1, healthcare careers share some attributes: they offer responsibility and opportunity with relatively limited training. Many careers also offer great earning potential, but the ways in which these careers are the same are much fewer than the ways in which they are different. Perhaps, after reading the job descriptions in Chapter 1, you knew immediately that working as a surgical technologist, for example, was the perfect choice for you. But for many people, the choice is not always perfectly clear.

If this is true for you, the self-evaluation that follows is an essential first step in finding the career that's right for you.

SELF-EVALUATION

Everybody has strengths and weaknesses, likes and dislikes. Understanding these aspects of your character will help you determine which career fits you best. It is very important to be as honest as you can when you conduct a self-evaluation. Your aim is to find the best career for you. There are no "right" answers in a self-evaluation. It is also important to create as complete a picture as you can.

Strengths and Weaknesses

To understand your strengths and weaknesses answer the following questions selecting very true, true, not very true, or not true.

I am compassionate when others are sick. _____

I am an upbeat, positive person. _____

I have a calm demeanor. _____

Angry or depressed people upset me. _____

Hospitals make me nervous. _____

The sight of blood doesn't bother me. _____

I am good at taking direction. _____

I work well under stress. _____

I am organized. _____

I pay close attention to detail. _____

I am good at solving problems. _____

I have good math skills. _____

I am good at working with machines. _____

I am physically fit. _____

I am good at clerical tasks. _____

These questions will help you get started thinking about your strengths and weaknesses. If you are not sure about an answer, for example, if you don't know if you work well under stress, try to think of the last time you were in a stressful situation. Did you handle it calmly and feel invigorated by the experience? Or, did you get frazzled and feel depleted by the experience? It often helps to imagine yourself in a situation, or, even better, remember a situation you've recently experienced, to help assess your particular strengths or weaknesses.

Once you've answered the questions, reread the job descriptions and the personal qualities for the careers in Chapter 1 and you can begin to narrow your search. Next, consider your likes and dislikes, which can be similar to strengths and weaknesses. For example, someone who is good at math will often enjoy solving math problems.

Likes and Dislikes

In order for a career to be right for you, it must be work that you enjoy. So, it is very important to have clear picture of your likes and dislikes. Answer the following questions selecting very true, true, not very true, or not true.

I enjoy caring for others. _____

I like to work with people. _____

I like variety in my work. _____

I like active work. _____

I like to have a set routine. _____

I enjoy office work. _____

I enjoy science and math. _____

I like to work alone. _____

I enjoy working on a team. _____

Use your answers to the questions above to narrow down your career choices. Again, it often helps to think about situations you've experienced to make an honest assessment of your likes and dislikes. For example, answer the following questions.

▶ What was the best job you've had (including any volunteer or part-time work)?

▶ What were the key characteristics of this work?

▶ What are your hobbies?

▶ What do you enjoy most about your hobbies?

▶ What clubs or organizations do you belong to?
▶ Why did you join these organizations?
▶ What were, or are, your favorite subjects in school?
▶ What subjects did, or do, you like least?

By considering both your strengths and weaknesses combined with your likes and dislikes you can begin to focus in on the right career for you. The questions listed above are only a very brief self-evaluation. For some people, a more extensive evaluation might be necessary. There are many resources that can help you make a career choice. They range from books and websites to professional career counselors.

Career Counseling Resources

Here are some of the best sources in print and online:

Career Development Manual: *www.adm.uwaterloo.ca/infocecs/CRC.*
The Career Key—A Free Public Service to Help People Make Sound Career Decisions: *www.ncsu.edu/careerkey.*
Mapping Your Future: *www.mapping-your-future.org.*
Online Career Counseling (free of charge): *www.onlinecareercounseling.com.*
Do What You Are: Discover the Perfect Career for You Through the Secrets of Personality Type. Paul D. Tieger and Barbara Barron-Tieger. (Little Brown, New York) 2001.
I Could Do Anything If I Only Knew What It Was: How to Discover What You Really Want and How to Get It. Barbara Sher. (DTP) 1995.
The Pathfinder: How to Choose or Change Your Career for a Lifetime of Satisfaction and Success. Nicholas Lore. (Fireside Publishing, New York) 1998.
What Color Is Your Parachute? 2002: A Practical Manual for Job-Hunters and Career-Changers. Richard Nelson Bolles. (Ten Speed Press, Berkeley) 2001.

If you are in high school, your guidance counselor can give you essential career advice. They make an assessment based on your transcript and through analyzing your performance on vocational interest and aptitude tests that examine your personal preferences and abilities in depth. If you are in college, a career counselor is often on staff to help you in the same manner as a guidance counselor. Some local offices of the state employment services affiliated with the federal employment service offer free counseling. A professional career counselor also offers many of the same services. You can search for a career counselor in your area online or in the telephone book. However, when paying for professional counseling, be sure that the person has valid credentials and a proven reputation. Counselors will not tell you what to do, but they can help guide you in your search for specialization.

Finally, one of the best tools to help you understand yourself and make decisions about your career is the people who know you well. Use the questions above to create a survey and poll the people who know you best—perhaps your parents, siblings, spouse, friends, or former employers. It is best to ask an assortment of people rather than relying on one person for career advice.

Next, you need to consider what experience you have already gained, and figure out how much training you are ready to pursue.

Where You Are Now

In order to consider your next step you need to have a clear picture of where you are now and how this will affect your career choices. Someone just finishing high school and making choices about attending college will have very different considerations than someone who is mid-career with a family and other obligations. Also, the level of training you elect to pursue will depend somewhat on what experience you have already gained. A person with a high school diploma and no job experience will have different training needs from a person who has a four-year college degree and some healthcare experience.

Level of Education

First consider what education you have already achieved.

▶ Do you have your high school diploma or equivalent?
▶ Have you taken math, science, and health classes?
▶ Do you have any college credits?
▶ If so, in what subjects do you have college credit?
▶ Have you taken your SATs or other college entrance exams?
▶ What are your scores?

Your answers to these questions will help you determine the level of training you are ready to pursue. In the recommended training section of the careers listed in chapter 1 you will find a description of the training programs and entrance requirements for each career. Of course, you can pursue any career profiled in this book, but your starting point may determine how much additional training will be required.

Personal Circumstances

Your personal circumstances will also affect how much training you want (and are able) to pursue. Answer these questions to help determine how much time and money you can commit to following your new career.

▶ Can you go to school full time or do you need to continue to work?
▶ Do you have money saved that you can use to cover the cost of attending school?
▶ Are you responsible for caring for children or other loved ones?
▶ How will this affect your training plans?
▶ What are your financial obligations?
▶ How do you plan to meet your financial obligations while you attend school?
▶ Can you travel or relocate to attend school or must you attend a program near your home?

A certificate can take three to six months to a year, an associate degree requires two years of training, and a bachelor's degree takes four years. The cost of attending these programs will increase relative to the length of the program. While there is financial aid that can help you meet the cost of tuition, which is covered in detail in Chapter 4, you must also consider the cost of not working while you are getting your training. Use your answers to the questions above to determine how much training you are willing, or able, to pursue.

Yet, you must balance any limits on the level of training you want seek with your career goals and ambitions. Some careers offer greater opportunities for advancement and better earning potential than others, and there is often a correlation between training and opportunity. Careers with relatively easy entrance requirements will generally offer fewer chances for advancement and will have lower earning potential.

Next you must consider where you want your career to take you and add that to the picture you have created so far.

Where You Want to Be

One of the most important steps in making a career decision is to consider what you want from work—not only from your entry-level job, but from your career in the long term. People have very different needs and ambitions, and they can be just as important as strengths and weaknesses in determining the right career for you.

Answer the following questions selecting very true, true, not very true, or not true.

I want to earn a high salary. _____

I am the primary earner in my household. _____

My career is an important priority in my life. _____

I want a career that allows me to have increasing responsibility. _____

I want to have a higher level position in five years. _____

Someday, I would like to supervise others. _____

I am willing to pursue more education to advance my career. _____

I am willing to postpone other life goals while I focus on my career. _____

Your answers to these questions should help you determine if you want a career with more opportunity and earning potential, remembering that these careers require a greater investment, or if you are more interested in career that you can enter with relative ease and will still find very satisfying. Of course, keep in mind that a career is a lifelong process. Many of the careers profiled in this book that have relatively easy entrance requirements are excellent stepping-stones to other healthcare careers.

You have begun to get a sense of the right career for you, but to make certain of your choice, you need to learn more about the job you've chosen. The descriptions in Chapter 1 are a great beginning, but they are necessarily brief. Here are some strategies for learning more about the career you would like to pursue.

RESEARCHING YOUR CAREER

When you have found a career that you think is right for you, you are ready to do some research. A career decision can be very important and it always helps to have more information.

Talk to People

One of the best ways to learn about a job is to talk to people who are already in a career. You can do this informally or you can conduct more formal informational interviews. First, ask yourself: Do I know someone or have a friend who knows someone who works in this field? If you do not have an immediate contact, you might have to be creative about your contacts.

The networking section in Chapter 5 has important tips about finding and expanding your contacts when you are looking for your first job. These tips also apply to finding people to talk to *before* you embark on a new career.

When you have contacted several people who you can talk to about your career choice, here are some questions that can help you learn if you're on the right track with your career choice:

▶ What is a typical day like for you?

▶ What do you like most about your work?

▶ What don't you like about your job?

▶ Do you think you will continue in this career?

▶ Why or why not?

▶ How did you get started in this career?

▶ Has it been what you expected?

▶ If you could have another career in healthcare, what would you be?

▶ Why?

▶ What personal traits help you succeed in this career?

▶ What do you think of the future for this career?

Try to talk to several people in your career choice. Does the job these people describe sound like the career you have in mind? Do you think you have a lot in common with the people with whom you've spoken? Remember that people often have mixed views on their work, but consider whether the overall picture sounds appealing to you.

Professional Publications and Websites

You can also learn a lot about your chosen career by reading professional publications and visiting websites dedicated to your career. In the appendices to this book, you will find a comprehensive list of resources for the careers profiled in Chapter 1. Through these resources, you can learn about trends in the career and employment issues as well as get a general feel for the profession.

To find more resources for the career of your choice, you can visit the Bureau of Labor Statistics online at www.bls.org. At this site, you can search for a specific job title and find a comprehensive job description as well as links to professional associations.

Your local library can also be a great resource. Visit the reference librarian and ask him or her how to find information about the career in which you are interested. The librarian will be able to point you to numerous resources including career guides, occupational handbooks, and other references that will help you learn if you've found the right career for you.

LEARNING MORE ABOUT TRAINING

Two important questions to have in mind when you research your career are what training is absolutely *necessary* and what training is *recommended*. Also keep in mind that the answer to this question may vary from state to state and even from one local area to another.

For example, you learn from your research that certification is required to be a surgical technologist in your state. But you may also learn that in order to get hired as a surgical technologist, you really need to have an associate's degree and to pass the national licensing exam. This information will be very important when you make your decision about training program.

You may even find in your research that you want to work in a particular hospital or practice. In this case, you can find out exactly what training you will need to get hired. In the next chapter you will learn all about training programs and how to select the best program for your training needs.

THE INSIDE TRACK

Who:	Crystal Dailey
What:	Health Information Technician
Where:	Omaha, Nebraska

INSIDER'S STORY

I didn't have a plan after high school. I wasn't ready for college, but the kinds of jobs that are open to people without a degree were limited (this is even more true now!). A friend of mine had a job as a home health aide, and she got me into a three-week training program and got me a position with her agency. I liked being involved with healthcare, but after a couple of years, I started to feel like I was burning out. Being a home health aide was isolating, because I worked by myself a lot of the time and didn't have coworkers with me to help blow off steam.

I didn't want to leave the healthcare field completely, so I went back to school and earned an associate's degree as a Health Information Technician from a community college in my area. This is the first job I've had as a technician, and I have been here for almost a year. Basically, my job is to maintain patient records, enter new information into our computer system, and code procedures electronically so that we can submit bills to insurance companies. I start files for new patients, make sure that we have all of the paperwork we need, and sometimes check with patients or doctors to clarify or get more information.

I find that this position suits me well because I've always been a stickler for detail! It bothers me to see even the smallest thing out of place—that's the degree of organization that's required to do a job like this efficiently. I work in a small clinic and we are understaffed, so another technician and I really do the work of three people, and it's important to keep on top of things and not let them get out of hand. It can be overwhelming sometimes; we get really busy with all of the incoming paperwork and requests for records. But it helps to think of every piece of paper as being attached to a person. That way, I remember that the work I do really affects someone's treatment. It's nice to help people, even in a way that is less direct than when I worked in home care.

My advice to someone considering a career in healthcare is that there's a wide variety of things to do in this field. When I decided to quit doing home care, I was tempted to start doing something completely different. But my experience turned out to be really useful; for example, I had an edge over the people in my classes who were fresh out of high school because I was familiar with healthcare terms and procedures. There are all kinds of options and different ways of helping people get the care they need, and whether you are right in there, helping someone eat or dress, or behind the scenes, making sure that insurance or Medicare will pay for them to see a doctor, you can be instrumental in helping people lead healthier, more comfortable lives.

CHAPTER three

ALL ABOUT TRAINING PROGRAMS

THIS CHAPTER IS all about getting the training you need for your future in healthcare. Now that you have decided which healthcare career you want to pursue, you need to make still more choices about getting the right training. In this chapter you will learn how to select the best program for your needs—from certificate programs through four-year degrees. You will see courses from several training programs across the country, so you can get an idea of what types of classes are required. There are tips for getting the most out of your training, from study strategies to career counseling advice. You will also learn about certification exams— what they are, why they are important, and how you can prepare for them.

THE IMPORTANCE OF TRAINING

As you have learned in your research so far, most jobs in the healthcare field, especially those jobs that involve direct patient treatment or operating equipment, require a period of training in a clinical setting so you can gain knowledge of hospital or physician office procedures. Requirements for entering your field of choice will most likely include the completion of a training program, such as obtaining some kind of certificate or associate degree. Even if certification is not a direct requirement in your chosen field, most employers prefer to hire candidates with some level of training and proven knowledge in their field.

Ideally, when you enter a training program you have already made a choice about your ultimate career goal. Not only will this ensure that you are getting the right training for the job, but it will also help you succeed in school. Particularly when you are a returning student with other responsibilities—a family, a job, and bills to pay—school can be challenging. If you know exactly what you are trying to achieve, you will be better motivated to face the pressures and demands of completing a training program.

While it's important to set goals for your career, getting training in the healthcare field should open doors for you not lock you into one job. The skills that you acquire in your healthcare training program will be applicable to many different jobs—whether you do the same job but in a different environment, or if you use your training and work experience as a launching pad for getting even more training to achieve a higher status and salary. As you have already learned there is a growing need for trained healthcare workers, and the training you acquire will prepare you for a bright future with countless possibilities.

MAKING DECISIONS ABOUT TRAINING

When you have decided on the career you want to pursue, picking the right training program should be fairly easy. However, if you are still not sure of which career is right for you, learning about the required training may help you come to a decision. When making a decision about where to obtain your training you need to answer several questions:

- ▶ Can I obtain training near where I currently live?
- ▶ What are the costs of the training program?
- ▶ What kind of financial aid can I receive from the school? Can I receive enough financial aid to attend a larger college or university?
- ▶ How much will tuition, books, and tools cost?
- ▶ What are the entrance requirements and am I qualified to apply?
- ▶ Can I attend school part-time?
- ▶ Is the school I plan to attend accredited?
- ▶ What special benefits does the program offer?
- ▶ Who are the instructors and what are their credentials?

Your budget and the cost of the training program will determine whether you should work part time and go to school part time, apply for financial aid, or participate in work-study, and whether you can afford a community college, a private college, or a state university.

You also will need to determine whether you can afford to relocate. A school offering training in your chosen field may be in your state but not in your town. Can you afford moving expenses? Can you afford a place of your own? Does the school have dormitories where you may live at a lower price? (Most small schools do not.) If you want to attend an out-of-state community college, in many cases your tuition will double. Before you apply to any school, be sure to visit and find out if it fits your needs.

The Right Location

There are many programs from which to choose. You can obtain healthcare training in almost every part of the country. So you must first decide where you want to obtain your training. In the back of this book you will find a list of training programs in each state. This list is not complete but it is a good starting point.

You can also find out about programs in your area or state by searching on the web. Some good sites for finding training programs are:

▶ Think College
www.ed.gov/thinkcollege
Run by the Department of Education, this site offers information on paying for college using government sources. It also has a page dedicated to returning students with a directory of colleges and information on applying. Its directory of U.S. community colleges will be especially useful for locating affordable healthcare programs.
▶ Peterson's College Channel
www.petersons.com
A comprehensive database of schools with Peterson's Collegequest, which allows for customized searches, including by field of study.
▶ Embark.com
www.embark.com

A searchable database of U.S. colleges including a career and technical school channel. This site allows you to apply to your school of choice online.

▶ Collegeboard.com

www.collegeboard.com

From the creators of the SAT placement test, this site offers tools for applying to college—including planning, test taking, finding the right college, and getting into and paying for college.

▶ College Is Possible

www.collegeispossible.org

A collection of colleges and universities providing information on paying for, preparing for, and choosing the right college.

The following books will also help you find programs in your area.

Peterson's Vocational and Technical Schools: West, 5th edition
Peterson's Vocational and Technical Schools: East, 4th edition

Two important things to keep in mind when you are deciding on where you want to go to school are the costs associated with moving. These costs include moving expenses, potentially increased living expenses in a new area, as well as the personal costs of moving such as leaving behind family and friends and adjusting to new surroundings. The other financial consideration is tuition. At most community colleges, out-of-state students pay almost twice as much as in-state students.

On the other hand, if you are considering a move to a new city or even a new state, it can be beneficial to attend school where you ultimately want to live. Many programs in healthcare require that students work in a local hospital or healthcare facility as part of their training. This can be a great first step to getting a job when you graduate. As a student you will begin to make connections—through your teachers and through the work you do as part of your education—in the local healthcare community. These connections can be an important part of your job search when you graduate.

Financial Considerations

Tuition for healthcare programs can vary a great deal. When narrowing down your choice of schools you need to take into account some financial questions. Some of these questions you have already considered when deciding where you want to go to school. Where you attend school will affect your tuition status—whether you are in-state or out-of-state. It will also affect your living expenses while you attend school.

When you are researching schools, find out what the tuition and fees are for the schools you are considering. Tuition is the cost of taking classes—some schools charge one tuition rate for the semester regardless of the exact number of credits, while other schools have a tuition rate per credit. You should also be aware of any fees that you will be required to pay. Fees cover all non-tuition expenses such as activity fees, student insurance, and lab fees (these can be quite expensive for some healthcare courses). Another item to consider in your financial calculations is the cost of textbooks and supplies.

Also look into any scholarships that the schools you are considering offer. You may be eligible for a full scholarship in which all your tuition and fees are covered. Find out if the school offers work-study options or any other financial aid. You will find out much more about financial aid in Chapter 4.

Entrance Requirements

Next you must consider the entrance requirements of the program you want to attend. Every school has certain standards that students must meet before they can enroll. For many community colleges and technical programs, if you meet the entrance requirements you can enroll. However, some programs are competitive, and is only some of the students who apply to the school are accepted.

Most programs will require that you are a high school graduate or that you have obtained a high school equivalency degree. Some may require that students have achieved a certain grade point average, say a 2.5 or better. Your performance in related courses, such as biology or health, might also affect your chances of admission.

Other criteria used in admitting applicants to programs include the Standard Achievement Test (SAT), which you may have taken in high school, the American College Test (ACT), other reading, writing, or science placement tests, recommendations and personal statements, and exams specific to certain fields, such as the Nursing School Entrance Exam or the Pharmacy College Admissions Test (PCAT).

Some schools also require a physical and blood work to check for contagious diseases. Students also may have to purchase health insurance if they are not already covered. The school should offer a liability or malpractice insurance policy at a small fee to students and explain the coverage.

Once you are accepted into a program, some schools will require you to complete an entrance exam such as the Science Placement Test (SPT), the Hobbit Exam, or the College Placement Test (CPT) to determine your placement in courses. These tests evaluate your reading, writing, and math skills. If, for example, you score low in math and high in science, you may be placed in a remedial math course such as Math 099 for review before you take Math 101.

Some schools also require Allied Health Entrance Exams such as the Allied Health Aptitude Test (AHAT) for entrance into community college healthcare programs and the Allied Health Profession Aptitude Test (AHPAT) for entrance into four-year colleges. These tests help identify qualified applicants by measuring general academic abilities and scientific knowledge.

Quality of the Program

Once you have narrowed down a list that includes schools that: (1) offer the courses you need to prepare for your chosen career; (2) are in the place where you want to study; (3) you can afford; and (4) have entrance requirements that you can meet, then you can select the best schools from among your list.

First, and most important, you must find out if the program you want to attend is *accredited*. This means that it has met certain national standards and has been approved by an accrediting agency. Graduating from an *accredited* program is a requirement for most state and national licenses in healthcare. It is usually easy to find out if a program is accredited because schools are proud of their accreditation. However, if the school brochures and website do not include a notice of accreditation, you can contact the accrediting organizations directly. These agencies can tell you if the program you are considering is accredited.

Many agencies accredit programs in every field of the healthcare industry. Don't be overwhelmed by the number of accrediting associations. Just be sure your targeted school lists one or more of them as its accrediting agency.

For example, the American Association of Medical Assistants (AAMA) Curriculum Review Board (CRB) assesses the quality of programs seeking accreditation for medical assistant technology. It then advises the Council on Accreditation and Unit Recognition (CAUR) of the Commission on Accreditation for Allied Health Education Programs (CAAHEP) as to whether the program should be accredited.

The Commission on Accreditation of Allied Health Education Programs (CAAHEP) and the Accrediting Bureau of Health Education Schools (ABHES) are both recognized by the U.S. Department of Education for accrediting such programs. For a list of associations that maintain lists or directories of accredited programs, see Appendix A under *Accrediting Bodies for Healthcare Education Programs*.

Next, you should find out about classroom size and teachers' credentials. The teacher-to-student ratio is an important factor in determining the quality of your education—the smaller the class size the more individual attention each student will receive. Also read about the faculty: where did they receive their training and what professional experience do they have? The program should include some faculty members with advanced degrees (MSW, MBA, Ph.D., and so on) and some with significant experience in the working world (at least five to seven years). Also, the faculty should be accessible for student conferences.

The placement rate for graduates is another important measure of the quality of a program, and when considering a school, whether small or large, you should ask about it. Many schools offer free placement services for the working lifetime of their graduates. If the graduates of a program go on to find employment and enjoy success in their field, then you can assume that they received good training and career placement support from the program.

Finally, learn about the facilities offered at the school. Particularly if you are entering a technical field such as surgical technologist or radiologic technician, you want to learn on the most up-to-date equipment and make sure that as a student you will have adequate access to the equipment. Many healthcare programs have a lab requirement and you will get the most out of a program that offers state of the art equipment.

FINDING OUT ABOUT PROGRAMS

You may be wondering how you will find all this detailed information. Your first step is to request literature from the schools on your narrowed-down list—their brochures and catalog. These will help answer your basic questions as you further narrow down your choices.

Next, you should make an appointment with an admissions officer. This person can answer the more specific questions you have about the program itself and the admission requirements. Ideally, you should have a face-to-face meeting. This will allow you to visit the school at the same time.

Visiting the school you plan to attend is the best way to get a feel for the program. When you visit, you can arrange to sit in on some classes. You may also be able to make an appointment to meet with a teacher in the program, and even with some students who are currently attending. Make sure you take a look at the classrooms and the labs. You might also visit the library and the career counseling center.

TYPES OF TRAINING PROGRAMS

Educational requirements for the health occupations discussed in this book generally range from three- to six-month or one-year certificate programs to two years of college. Training for entry-level positions is offered in high schools, vocational–technical centers, community colleges, universities, hospitals, nursing homes, and the Armed Forces, depending on the type of program you are seeking. Most programs provide both classroom and clinical instruction.

High School Programs for Non-Graduated Students

If you haven't graduated from high school or received your GED yet, and you are under 20 years old, your area school district may have a Youth Apprenticeship program designed just for you. It is also for students in grades 10 to 12 who want to pursue healthcare careers. Apprenticeship programs work with different governmental and social service agencies to offer students structured school- and work-based learning that leads to a high school diploma, post-secondary credential, or certificate. Healthcare youth apprentice programs work with hospitals to open avenues to higher education and certifiable occupations.

School districts offer other programs such as Tech Prep, Cooperative Education, Internships, Explorations in Technology, and Micro Society. These examples may vary from state to state, but they all offer educational skills to apply in real-life healthcare employment situations. You can learn more about these programs by calling your local school district, or if you are already a student, by speaking with your guidance counselor.

Certificate Programs

Certificate programs are usually three- to six-month or six-month to one-year programs, and graduates receive a certificate of completion. Entrance requirements generally include a high school diploma or its equivalent, and in some cases entrance exams are required. Courses combine classroom theory with clinical instruction. Certificate programs are usually conducted without breaks, unlike associate degree programs, which generally follow a semester schedule with breaks between the semesters.

Nursing Assistant Sample Curriculum

The curriculum for certificate programs varies among schools and programs. Here is the curriculum for a certificate course for nursing assistants offered at Green River Community College in Auburn, Washington. The certificate course is designed to prepare nursing assistants for competency as outlined by federal and Washington State curricula.

Course Number	Course Title	Credits
Nurse 100	Nutrition	3
Nurse 104	Nursing 1—Fundamentals	6
Nurse 105	Community Lab 1	4
Nurse 106	Nursing 2	8
Nurse 107	Nursing 2—Community Lab 2	8
Nurse 116	Nursing Issues and Delivery System	3
English 108	Medical Terminology	2

Source: Green River Community College, www.grcc.ctc.edu.

Full-time tuition (10 to 18 credits) at Green River Community College is $547 per semester for in-state students. For non-residents, full-time tuition is $2,153 per semester. Students also pay between $30 and $50 in fees each semester.

Sonography Certificate Sample Curricula

Like many sonography programs, the Diagnostic Medical Sonography Training Program at Hudson Valley Community College in New York State is intended as additional training for people who have already achieved some secondary education in the healthcare field. Candidates who have completed a two-year healthcare training program that is patient-care related are eligible. Individuals who have completed a bachelor's degree (with eight credits of Anatomy and Physiology included) are also eligible for the program. Direct patient care experience is necessary. The program is one year long and students take the following classes:

First Semester

Course #	Title	Credits
03561	Diagnostic Sonography I	3
03575	Cross Sectional Anatomy of the Abdomen	2
03576	Cross Sectional Anatomy of OB-GYN	2

03581	Sonography Clinic I	8
	Semester Total	15
	Intersession Clinic* (two 40-hour weeks, as part of 03581)	

Second Semester

Course #	Title	Credits
03562	Diagnostic Sonography II	4
03577	Pathophysiology of the Abdomen	2
03578	Pathophysiology of OB-GYN	2
03582	Sonography Clinic II	8
	Semester Total	16

Summer Session

03583	Sonography Clinic III*	13

*Additional clinical experience at assigned hospital is required to qualify for National Certifying Exam (ARDMS).

Source: Hudson Valley Community College, www.hvcc.edu.

Tuition at Hudson Valley Community College is $98 per credit for full-time, in-state students. The fees are $110 per semester, and there is an additional lab fee that ranges from $10 to $200 per lab course.

Associate Degree Programs

An associate degree program requires two academic or two calendar years. Entrance requirements include a high school diploma or a GED, and some programs require college prep courses. Most associate degree programs require entrance and placement exams. In many associate degree programs, half the required courses are in liberal arts and half are in the major. Courses in the major combine classroom theory with clinical practice in extended care facilities, hospitals, and community agencies.

Generally, an associate degree will lead to a job with higher pay and greater advancement opportunity than a certificate. Associate degrees are offered by community colleges and junior colleges. Community colleges are usually public and have very reasonable tuition rates. Junior colleges are private and can have tuition rates that are comparable to four-year private colleges.

Medical Assistant Associate Degree Sample Curriculum

This program offered at Long Technical College in Phoenix, Arizona, is a two-year program to prepare student with the knowledge, technical skills, and work habits required for an entry-level position as a medical assistant working under the direction of the physician in private or group practices, clinics, and other medical facilities. Graduates may choose to specialize in front or back office duties, or diversify and do both. Upon successful completion of the program, graduates will be awarded an Associate of Occupational Studies.

Associate of Occupational Studies in Medical Assisting program takes 64 academic weeks to complete for day students, or 78 academic weeks for night students. All students must complete the program with 97.5 quarter credit hours. Courses offered in the program include:

Course Number	Course Name	Credit Hours
MA 04	Professional Development	2.0
MA 05	Keyboarding & Computer Basics	2.0
MA 06	Medisoft	2.0
MA 07	WordPerfect	2.0
MA 08	Communication for Health Professionals	2.0
MA 09	Medical Office Management I	3.0
MA 10	Medical Office Bookkeeping	3.0
MA 11	Medical Office Insurance I	3.0
MA 12	Medical Back Office A	5.0
MA 13	Medical Back Office B	6.5
MA 14	Medical Back Office C	6.5
MA 15	Medical Back Office D	5.0
MA 18	Externship I	5.0
MA 16	Medical Psychology I	4.0
MA 17	Medical Psychology II	4.0
MA 19	Medical Office Insurance II	6.5
SM 119	Nutrition & Pharmacology	6.5
MA 22	Medical Office Management II	6.0
MA 24	Medical Office English	3.0
MA 25	Medical Research & Writing	3.0
SM 110	Musculoskeletal Physiology, Fractures, and Casting	6.0

SM 118	Sterile Techniques	6.5
MA 26	Externship II	5.0

Source: Long Technical College, www.longtechnicalcollege.com.

Because Long is a private technical college, it has higher tuition and fees than you would find at a community college. The total tuition and fee cost of the two-year program including all fees, tuition, textbooks, and supplies is $17,746. This does not include commuting or other personal costs. The tuition and fee costs are broken down as follows:

Registration Fee	$100
Application Fee	$25
Tuition 1st Academic Year	$7,520
Tuition 2nd Academic Year	$8,080
Textbooks 1st Academic Year	$265
Textbooks 2nd Academic Year	$280
Lab Fees/Supplies 1st Academic Year	$520
Lab Fees/Supplies 2nd Academic Year	$540
Insurance	$184
Uniforms	$232

Respiratory Technologist Sample Curriculum

Tallahassee Community College in Tallahassee, Florida, offers a two-year program in respiratory care that leads to an associate in science degree. The program is designed to prepare students for the examinations offered by the National Board for Respiratory Therapy. Graduates have the skills to become Registered Respiratory Therapists who can perform competently in the responsibilities of helping to diagnose and care for persons with cardiopulmonary diseases.

The six-semester program of study in respiratory care is accredited by the Committee on Allied Health Education and Accreditation (CAHEA) of the American Medical Association. The program includes the following courses:

First Year Courses

(46 Credit Hours)

CHM 1032 General Chemistry for Health (3)

BSC 2085 Anatomy and Physiology (3)

BSC 2085L Anatomy and Physiology Lab (1)

RET 1026 Fundamentals of Respiratory Care (3)

RET 1026L Fundamentals of Respiratory Care Lab (1)

RET 1483 Assessment I (1)

RET 1874 Clinical Practice I (1)

RET 1874L Clinical Practice I Lab (1)

RET 2485 Cardio-Pulmonary Physiology (4)

RET 1350 Cardio-Pulmonary Pharmacology (4)

HSC 2531 Medical Terminology (3)

RET 1450 Assessment II (1)

RET 1875 Clinical Practice II (2)

RET 1434 Assessment III (1)

RET 2876 Clinical Practice III (1)

RET 2264 Advanced Procedures (3)

RET 2264L Advanced Procedures Lab (1)

RET 2027 Instrumentation (1)

HSC 1651 Ethics for Health Care (1)

CGS 1141 Computer Literacy for Health Sciences (2)

RET 1293 Cardio-Pulmonary Disease (4)

MGS 1106 Mathematics I for Liberal Arts (3)

Second Year Courses

(30 Credit Hours)

RET 2534 Assessment IV (1)

ENC 1101 College Composition (3)

RET 2714 Pediatrics & Neonatology (2)

RET 2714L Pediatrics & Neonatology Lab (1)

RET 2442 Hemodynamics (2)

RET 2442L Hemodynamics Lab (1)

RET 2877 Clinical Practice IV (2)

RET 2414 Pulmonary Function (2)

RET 2418 Assessment V (1)

RET 2878 Clinical Practice V (2)
RET 2879 Clinical Practice V (2)
MCB 2004 Microbiology (3)
MCB 2004 Microbiology Lab (1)
Social Science Elective (3)

Source: Tallahassee Community College, www.tcc.cc.fl.us.

The tuition at Tallahassee Community College is $50 per credit hour for in-state students and $187 per credit hour for out-of-state students. Additional fees include $10 per semester student services fee and additional lab fees.

Baccalaureate Programs

The bachelor degree program combines major courses with general education in a four-year curriculum in a college or university. You may be admitted to your major program as a freshman or after completing one or two years of general education at the school or another institution. If, for example, you go to a small college or technical school to become a surgical technician and earn an associate degree, and then later decide that you want to earn a higher degree and level of salary, you can apply the credits you have already earned toward your bachelor's degree.

A high school diploma or its equivalent (GED) is required for admission, and placement exams, SAT scores, ACT scores, and an acceptable high school GPA may be required. Entrance requirements may be more competitive than for shorter training programs. You may have to take a higher level of tests to enter the specific major area, such as the Allied Health Aptitude Test (AHAT). Because a bachelor's degree requires at least four years of school if you don't already have some schooling, you may, like most students, require some financial aid. However, you should not write off a college education for financial reasons. Remember, there are scholarships and loans, plus a number of other ways to help pay for college. (See Chapter 4 for details about financial aid.)

MAKING THE MOST OF YOUR TRAINING PROGRAM

When you have decided on the right school for you, applied, and been admitted to the program you will be well on your way to a rewarding career in healthcare. However, simply getting into a program and going to class is not enough. You have worked hard to get into your training program, and you will need to keep up the good work when you get there. Not only do you want to get good grades, but you will also begin building the network you will rely upon when you start to look for work.

During your training program you want to make a good impression on your instructors and the people you work with during the clinical portion of your training. These are the people who can give you recommendations and job leads when you graduate. It is important that you impress them with your abilities and your attitude when you are in school. Perhaps even more important, school is your chance to learn the skills necessary for your profession. Healthcare is a serious undertaking and when you work in healthcare you play an important role in the health and well being of your patients. You will want to get the best training you can so that you can do your job with confidence.

The rest of this chapter shows you how to maximize the learning process. Apply the tips listed below to get the most out of your training program.

How to Study for Exams

Remember studying for exams in high school? No matter what your IQ, studying is crucial to success in a training program, where the work is much tougher than in high school. However, don't let the word *exam* make you nervous. Exams are the instructor's way of finding out what you have learned and what you may need to review before going any further with assignments. If you have been keeping up with the work in class you should be prepared for the exam. Studying allow you to test your knowledge and to refresh your memory so that all the information you have learned during class will be available in your mind at exam time.

Some instructors will tell you to study at least two hours for each hour of class. This may seem difficult and time-consuming, but there are ways to make it easier, including reviewing your notes, reading appropriate textbook chapters, studying with others, and studying between classes. There is more information on these techniques later in the chapter.

If you remain on task in classes and labs and review steadily, you should have no problem with exams. Many exams are multiple choice, and the wrong answers will point you to the correct answer. Essay exams require you to write more detailed responses. It is helpful to know the format of the exam so you can study accordingly. An instructor will usually tell students what to expect on an exam.

For a multiple-choice test, you will probably focus more on memorizing terms and facts. And for an essay test you might work out responses to more procedural questions. During the test, it is essential to read the instructions carefully and listen to your instructor's directions.

How to Take Notes in Class

Taking good notes in class will help you to study after class. Listen attentively and try to write down the most important information. Many instructors indicate what you should write down and what is already in the book you will be studying. If an instructor writes anything on the board or on an overhead, you should write it down, too. Writing down too much information is better than writing too little, but be sure you are listening to the instructor as well as taking notes. You want to avoid transcribing the lecture. Try to pick out the main topic and the important facts.

Rewriting your notes from each class will help you sort out the needed information and reinforce the information discussed in class.

Studying with Other Students

Studying with other students is one of the best ways to learn. Teaching another person can help you to learn and remember the material yourself. Also, having someone quiz you or explain something that you don't understand can help you work through a topic with which you are having trouble. Create a study group or join one. Because everyone has particular strengths, a group can combine the best skills of each individual to the benefit of everyone.

Also, if you have to miss a class or your notes for a particular day are not very good, your study group can be a great resource. Of course, a study group is only effective if all the students attend class, take notes, and do the homework.

Getting to Know Your Instructor

The first thing you should do after entering a class is make an appointment to meet with the instructor so you can ask questions, get to know him or her, and find out what's expected of you. Each instructor is different and has different expectations. Also, if you have any special concerns or needs, you can inform the instructor ahead of time.

In the clinical classes, you may have the opportunity to get to know instructors personally while working directly with them. Many instructors work one-on-one with students in the most difficult part of the program to make sure they understand the procedures and instructions, become oriented, and really learn that procedure. Instructors may go with you to the hospital or clinic where you will receive additional clinical education.

Using the Career Planning and Placement Office

Most schools have a career planning and placement office. Make an appointment right away to meet with a counselor in your field so you can begin working on a plan for job hunting before your graduation or certificate release. Your counselor will help you build your resume, tell you about job prospects in your area of specialization, and perhaps set up a placement file that allows you to send resume information directly from the school.

Career centers offer a variety of career-advising activities, such as one-on-one sessions in which students and advisors discuss effective career decision-making preferences, interests, values, and other concerns. Establishing goals is an important part of these sessions. You can make an appointment at any time throughout your training program if you have questions about your future career. Other services offered may include a career services library, a videotape library, a career and life development workshop, an information line/job vacancy hotline, internship programs, student employment services, career days, workshops, and mock and on-campus interviews. Each school is different, so career placement programs and services will vary.

As you have read in this chapter, your training is one of the most important steps in getting your healthcare career started. It is an exciting time and something over which you have almost total control. If you do the research, you will find a program that is exactly suited to your needs and goals. And when you're in school, you can make the most of your program so that you will graduate as a top candidate in the field of your choice.

Many people think that finances are preventing them from achieving their dreams. What they may not realize is that you do not necessarily need to have money saved in order to get the training you need. The next chapter is all about finding financial aid for your education.

THE INSIDE TRACK

Who:	Therese Wilkes
What:	Physical Therapist Assistant
Where:	Queens, New York

INSIDER'S STORY

I'm a physical therapist assistant, and I work at a clinic run by a local non-profit group that provides services for children with cerebral palsy and their families. I work with a physical therapist, but our office employs a number of assistants and only two therapists, so I work independently a good deal of the time, consulting with the therapist on how patients respond and how the therapy is progressing. Cerebral palsy doesn't have a cure, so our treatments aim to maintain muscle strength and help the kids use braces and other aids.

I work a 40-hour week, but my hours vary a lot. The center is open seven days a week, and a lot of our clients are only able to come for treatment in the evenings or on weekends. Often, I will work a week of regular 9-to-5 shifts, followed by a week of shifts from 12 to 8. It was hard at first to get used to those hours, and to not always having a full weekend off, but I've adjusted to it.

I did have to have training to get this job. A lot of people confuse physical therapy assistants and aides—an assistant, like me, has been through a two-year training program and can take on more responsibility in the therapy setting. At our clinic, aides are involved with some parts of the actual therapy, but more often they are responsible for the administrative functions of the office, making appointments, and preparing the therapy area for sessions. I worked as an aide while I was in school, and that experience was helpful in getting this job also—having a practical knowledge of physical therapy in addition to the academic knowledge learned in a training program.

I've thought about becoming a certified therapist. I definitely enjoy what I do, but I don't know if I'm ready to commit to two more years of school to get my bachelor's degree, and then two more on top of that for a master's. For the time being, I'm content to stay where I am; I feel lucky to work in a place where I have a great deal of freedom and people trust me to make judgments about the therapy I administer.

To succeed in this field, you really have to enjoy people—and I don't mean the clichéd "people person." Working in a therapy setting requires you to not only interact well with patients, but to touch them and to really get in there, regardless of the condition of the body. It's important not only to not be at all squeamish, but to have a gentle, reassuring touch and a positive demeanor. You are helping patients fix themselves, so you need to be in tip-top shape—both physically and mentally.

CHAPTER four

FINANCING YOUR EDUCATION

IN CHAPTER 3 you learned how to find and succeed in the right training program for you. This chapter explains some of the many different types of financial aid available, gives you information on what financial records you will need to gather to apply for financial aid, and helps you through the process of applying for financial aid. (A sample financial aid form is included in Appendix C.) At the end of the chapter are listed many more resources that can help you find the aid you need.

YOU HAVE decided on a career in healthcare and you've chosen a training program. Now, you need a plan to finance your training. Perhaps you or your family have been saving for your education, and you've got the money to pay your way. Or maybe your employer offers some money to help its employees attend school. However, if you're like most students, you don't have enough to cover the cost of the training program you'd like to attend. Be assured that it is likely that you can qualify for some sort of financial aid, even if you plan to attend school only part-time.

Because there are many types of financial aid, and the millions of dollars given away or loaned are available through so many sources, the process of finding funding for your education can seem confusing. Read through this chapter carefully, and check out the many resources, including websites and publications, listed at the end of this chapter and in Appendix B. You will have a better understanding of where to look for financial aid, what you can qualify for, and how and when to apply.

Also take advantage of the financial aid office at the school you've chosen, or your guidance counselor if you're still in high school. These professionals can offer plenty of information, and can help to guide you through the process. If you're not in school, and haven't chosen a program yet, check the Internet. It's probably the best source for up-to-the-minute information, and almost all of it is free. There are a number of great sites at which you can fill out questionnaires with information about yourself and receive lists of scholarships and other forms of financial aid for which you may qualify. You can also apply for some types of federal and state aid online—you can even complete the Free Application for Federal Student Aid (FAFSA), the basic form that determines federal and state financial aid eligibility, online if you choose.

SOME MYTHS ABOUT FINANCIAL AID

The subject of financial aid is often misunderstood. Here are some of the most common myths:

Myth #1: All the red tape involved in finding sources and applying for financial aid is too confusing for me.
Fact: The whole financial aid process is a set of steps that are ordered and logical. Besides, several sources of help are available. To start, read this chapter carefully to get a helpful overview of the entire process and tips on how to get the most financial aid. Then, use one or more of the resources listed within this chapter and in the appendices for additional help. If you believe you will be able to cope with your training program, you will be able to cope with looking for the money to finance it—especially if you take the process one step at a time in an organized manner.

Myth #2: For most students, financial aid just means getting a loan and going into heavy debt, which isn't worth it, or working while in school, which will lead to burnout and poor grades.

Fact: Both the federal government and individual schools award grants and scholarships which a student doesn't have to pay back. It is also possible to get a combination of scholarships and loans. It's worth taking out a loan if it means attending the program you really want to attend, rather than settling for your second choice or not pursuing a career in your chosen field at all. As for working while in school, it's true that it is a challenge to hold down a full-time or even part-time job while in school. However, a small amount of work-study employment (10–12 hours per week) has been shown to actually improve academic performance, because it teaches students important time-management skills.

Myth #3: I can't understand the financial aid process because of all the unfamiliar terms and strange acronyms that are used.

Fact: While you will encounter an amazing number of acronyms and some unfamiliar terms while applying for federal financial aid, you can refer to the acronym list and glossary at the end of this chapter for quick definitions and clear explanations of the commonly used terms and acronyms.

Myth #4: Financial aid is for students attending academic colleges or universities. I'm going to a vocational training program so I won't qualify.

Fact: This is a myth that far too many people believe. The truth is, there is considerable general financial aid for which vocational students qualify. There are also grants and scholarships specifically designed for students in vocational programs. The financial aid you get may be less than that for longer, full-time programs, but it can still help you pay for a portion of your training program.

Myth #5: My family makes too much money (or I make too much money), so I shouldn't bother to apply for financial aid.

Fact: The formula used to calculate financial aid eligibility is complex and takes more into account than just your or your family's income. Also, some forms of financial aid—such as a PLUS Loan or an unsubsidized Stafford Loan—are available regardless of calculated financial need. The only way to be certain NOT to get financial aid is to not apply; don't shortchange yourself by not applying, even if you think you won't be eligible.

TYPES OF FINANCIAL AID

There are three categories of financial aid:

1. Grants and scholarships—aid that you don't have to pay back
2. Work-study—aid that you earn by working
3. Loans—aid that you have to pay back

Each of these types of financial aid will be examined in greater detail, so you will be able to determine which one(s) to apply for, and when and how to apply. Note that grants and scholarships are available on four levels: federal, state, school, and private.

Grants

Grants are normally awarded based on financial need. Even if you believe you won't be eligible based on your own or your family's income, don't skip this section. There are some grants awarded for academic performance and other criteria. The two most common grants, the Pell Grant and Federal Supplemental Educational Opportunity Grant (FSEOG), are both offered by the federal government.

Federal Pell Grants

Federal Pell Grants are based on financial need and are awarded only to undergraduate students who have not yet earned a bachelor's or professional degree. For many students, Pell Grants provide a foundation of financial aid to which other aid may be added. For the year 2001–2002, the maximum award was $3,750.00. You can receive only one Pell Grant in an award year, and you may not receive Pell Grant funds for more than one school at a time.

How much you get will depend not only on your Expected Family Contribution (EFC) but also on your cost of attendance, whether you're a full-time or part-time student, and whether you attend school for a full academic year or less. You can qualify for a Pell Grant even if you are only enrolled part time in a training program. You should also be aware that some private and school-based sources of financial aid will not consider your eligibility if you haven't first applied for a Pell Grant.

Federal Supplemental Educational Opportunity Grants (FSEOG)

Priority consideration for FSEOG funds is given to students receiving Pell Grants because the FSEOG program is based on exceptional financial need. An FSEOG is similar to a Pell Grant in that it doesn't need to be paid back.

If you are eligible, you can receive between $100 and $4,000 a year in FSEOG funds depending on when you apply, your level of need, and the funding level of the school you're attending. The FSEOG differs from the Pell Grant in that it is not guaranteed that every needy student will receive one because each school is only allocated a certain amount of FSEOG funds by the federal government to distribute among all eligible students. To have the best chances of getting this grant, apply for financial aid as early as you can after January 1 of the year in which you plan to attend school.

State Grants

State grants are generally specific to the state in which you or which your parents reside. If you and your parents live in the state in which you will attend school, you've got only one place to check. However, if you will attend school in another state, or your parents live in another state, be sure to check your eligibility with your state grant agency. Not all states allow their state grants to be used at out-of-state schools. There is a list of state agencies in Appendix A, including telephone numbers and websites, so you can easily find out if there is a grant for which you can apply.

Scholarships

Scholarships are often awarded for academic merit or for special characteristics (for example, ethnic heritage, personal interests, sports, parents' career, college major, geographic location) rather than financial need. As with grants, you do not pay your award money back. Scholarships may be offered from federal, state, school, and private sources.

The best way to find scholarship money is to use one of the free search tools available on the Internet. After entering the appropriate information about yourself, a search takes place which ends with a list of those prizes for which you are eligible. Try www.fastasp.org, which bills itself as the world's largest and oldest private sector scholarship database. A couple of other good sites for conducting searches are www.college-scholarships.com and www.gripvision.com.If you don't have easy access to the Internet, or want to expand your search, your high school guidance counselors or college financial aid officers also have plenty of information about available scholarship money. Also, check out your local library.

To find private sources of aid, spend a few hours in the library looking at scholarship and fellowship books or consider a reasonably priced (under $30) scholarship search service. See the Resources section at the end of this chapter to find contact information for search services and scholarship book titles.

Also, contact some or all of the professional associations for the program you're interested in attending; some offer scholarships, while others offer information about where to find scholarships. If you're currently employed, find out if your employer has scholarship funds available. If you're a dependent student, ask your parents and other relatives to check with groups or organizations they belong to as well as their employers to see if they have scholarship programs or contests. Investigate these popular sources of scholarship money:

- ▶ religious organizations
- ▶ fraternal organizations
- ▶ clubs (such as Rotary, Kiwanis, American Legion, Grange, or 4-H)
- ▶ athletic clubs
- ▶ veterans' groups (such as the Veterans of Foreign Wars)
- ▶ ethnic group associations
- ▶ unions
- ▶ local chambers of commerce

If you already know which school you will attend, check with a financial aid administrator (FAA) in the financial aid office to find out if you qualify for any school-based scholarships or other aid. Many schools offer merit-based aid for students with a high school GPA of a certain level or with a certain level of SAT scores in order to attract more students to their school. Check with your program's academic department to see if they maintain a bulletin board or other method of posting available scholarships.

While you are looking for sources of scholarships, continue to enhance your chances of winning one by participating in extracurricular events and volunteer activities. You should also obtain references from people who know you well and are leaders in the community, so you can submit their names and/or letters with your scholarship applications. Make a list of any awards you've received in the past or other honors that you could list on your scholarship application.

Hope Scholarship Credit

Eligible taxpayers may claim a federal income tax credit for tuition and fees up to a maximum of $1,500.00 per student (the amount is scheduled to be reindexed for inflation after 2002). The credit applies only to the first two years of postsecondary education, and students must be enrolled at least half-time in a program leading to a degree or a certificate. To find out more about the Hope Scholarship credit, log on to www.sfas.com.

Lifetime Learning Credit

Eligible taxpayers may claim a federal income tax credit for tuition and fees up to a maximum of $1,000 per student through the year 2002. After the year 2002, eligible taxpayers may claim a credit for tuition and fees up to a maximum of $2,000 per student (unlike the Hope Scholarship Credit, this amount will not be reindexed for inflation after 2002). The Lifetime Learning Credit is not limited to the first two years of postsecondary education; students in any year can be eligible, and there is no minimum enrollment requirement. For more information about the Lifetime Learning Credit, log on to www.sfas.com.

The National Merit Scholarship Corporation

This program offers about 5,000 students scholarship money each year based solely on academic performance in high school. If you are a high school senior with excellent grades and high scores on tests such as the ACT or SAT, ask your guidance counselor for details about this scholarship.

You may also be eligible to receive a scholarship from your state or school. Check with the higher education department of the relevant state or the financial aid office of the school you will attend.

Work-Study Programs

When applying to a college or university, you can indicate that you are interested in a work-study program. Their student employment office will have the most information about how to earn money while getting your education. Work options include the following:

- ▶ on- or off-campus
- ▶ part-time or almost full-time
- ▶ school- or nationally based
- ▶ in some cases, in your program of study (to gain experience) or not (just to pay the bills)
- ▶ for money to repay student loans or to go directly toward educational expenses

If you are interested in school-based employment, the student employment office can give you details about the types of jobs offered (which can range from giving tours of the campus to prospective students to working in the cafeteria to helping other students in a student services office) and how much they pay.

You should also investigate the Federal Work-Study (FWS) program, which can be applied for on the Free Application for Federal Student Aid (FAFSA). The FWS program provides jobs for undergraduate and graduate students with financial need, allowing them to earn money to help pay education expenses. It encourages community service work and provides hands-on experience related to your course of study, when available. The amount of the FWS award depends on:

- ▶ when you apply (apply early!)
- ▶ your level of need
- ▶ the FWS funds available at your particular school

FWS salaries are the current federal minimum wage or higher, depending on the type of work and skills required. As an undergraduate, you will be paid by the hour (a graduate student may receive a salary), and you will receive the money directly from your school; you cannot be paid by commission or fee. The awards are not transferable from year to year, and not all schools have work-study programs in every area of study.

An advantage of working under the FWS program is that your earnings are exempt from FICA taxes if you are enrolled full-time and are working less than half-time. You will be assigned a job on-campus, in a private nonprofit organization, or a public agency that offers a public service. You may provide a community service relating to fire or other emergency service if your school has such a program. Some schools have agreements with private, for-profit companies, if the work demands your fire or other emergency skills. The total wages you earn in each year cannot exceed your total FWS award for that year and you cannot work more than twenty hours per week. Your financial aid administrator (FAA) or the direct employer must consider your class schedule and your academic progress before assigning your job.

For more information about National Work Study programs, visit the Corporation for National Service website (www.cns.gov) or contact:

▶ **National Civilian Community Corps (NCCC)**—This AmeriCorps program is an 11-month residential national service program intended for 18–24-year-olds. Participants receive $4,725.00 for college tuition or to help repay education loan debt. Contact: National Civilian Community Corps, 1100 Vermont Avenue NW, Washington, DC 20525, 800-94-ACORPS.

▶ **Volunteers in Service to America (VISTA)**—VISTA is a part of ACTION, the deferral domestic volunteer agency. This program offers numerous benefits to college graduates with outstanding student loans. Contact: VISTA, 1000 Wisconsin Ave. NW, Washington, DC 20007, Tel: 800-424-8867.

If you are already working in the field in which you intend to go to school, your employer may help you pay for job-related courses. Check with your employer for details.

Student Loans

Although scholarships, grants, and work-study programs can help to offset the costs of higher education, they usually don't give you enough money to pay your way entirely. Most students who can't afford to pay for their entire education rely at least in part on student loans. The largest single source of these loans—and for all money for students—is the federal government. However, you can also find loan money from your state, school, and/or private sources.

Try these sites for information about U.S. government programs:

www.fedmoney.org
This site explains everything from the application process (you can actually download the applications you will need), eligibility requirements, and the different types of loans available.

www.finaid.org
Here, you can find a calculator for figuring out how much money your education will cost (and how much you will need to borrow), get instructions for filling out the necessary forms, and even information on the various types of military aid (which will be detailed in the next chapter).

www.ed.gov/offices/OSFAP/students
This is the Federal Student Financial Aid Homepage. The FAFSA (Free Application for Federal Student Aid) can be filled out and submitted online. You can find a sample FAFSA in Appendix C, to help familiarize yourself with its format.

www.students.gov
This bills itself as the "student gateway to the U.S. government" and is run as a cooperative effort under the leadership of the Department of Education. You can find information about financial aid, community service, military service, career development, and much more.

You can also get excellent detailed information about different federal sources of education funding by sending away for a copy of the U.S. Department of Education's publication, *The Student Guide*. Write to: Federal Student Aid Information Center, P.O. Box 84, Washington, DC 20044, or call 800-4FED-AID.

Listed below are some of the most popular federal loan programs:

Federal Perkins Loans

A Perkins Loan has the lowest interest (currently, it's 5%) of any loan available for both undergraduate and graduate students, and is offered to students with exceptional financial need. You repay your school, which lends the money to you with government funds.

Depending on when you apply, your level of need, and the funding level of the school, you can borrow up to $4,000 for each year of undergraduate study. The total amount you can borrow as an undergraduate is $20,000 if you have completed two years of undergraduate study; otherwise, you can borrow a maximum of $8,000.

The school pays you directly by check or credits your tuition account. You have nine months after you graduate (provided you were continuously enrolled at least half-time) to begin repayment, with up to ten years to pay off the entire loan.

PLUS Loans (Parent Loan for Undergraduate Students)

PLUS Loans enable parents with good credit histories to borrow money to pay the education expenses of a child who is a dependent undergraduate student enrolled at least half-time. Your parents must submit the completed forms to your school.

To be eligible, your parents will be required to pass a credit check. If they don't pass, they might still be able to receive a loan if they can show that extenuating circumstances exist or if someone who is able to pass the credit check agrees to co-sign the loan. Your parents must also meet citizenship requirements and not be in default on any federal student loans of their own.

The yearly limit on a PLUS Loan is equal to your cost of attendance minus any other financial aid you receive. For instance, if your cost of attendance is $10,000 and you receive $5,000 in other financial aid, your parents could borrow up to, but no more than, $5,000. The interest rate varies, but is not to exceed 9% over the life of the loan. Your parents must begin repayment while you're still in school. There is no grace period.

Federal Stafford Loans

Stafford Loans are low-interest loans that are given to students who attend school at least half-time. The lender is the U.S. Department of Education for schools that participate in the Direct Lending program and a bank or credit union for schools that do not participate in the Direct Lending program. Stafford Loans fall into one of two categories:

Subsidized loans are awarded on the basis of financial need. You will not be charged any interest before you begin repayment or during authorized periods of deferment. The federal government subsidizes the interest during these periods.

Unsubsidized loans are not awarded on the basis of financial need. You will be charged interest from the time the loan is disbursed until it is paid in full. If you allow the interest to accumulate, it will be capitalized—that is, the interest will be added to the principal amount of your loan, and additional interest will be based upon the higher amount. This will increase the amount you have to repay.

There are many borrowing limit categories to these loans, depending on whether you get an unsubsidized or subsidized loan, which year in school you're enrolled, how long your program of study is, and if you're independent or dependent. You can have both kinds of Stafford Loans at the same time, but the total amount of money loaned at any given time cannot exceed $23,000 for a dependent undergraduate student and $46,000 as an independent undergraduate student (of which not more than $23,000 can be in subsidized Stafford Loans). The interest rate varies, but will never exceed 8.25%. An origination fee for a Stafford Loan is approximately 3% or 4% of the loan, and the fee will be deducted from each loan disbursement you receive. There is a six-month grace period after graduation before you must start repaying the loan.

State Loans

Loan money is also available from state governments. In Appendix A you will find a list of the agencies responsible for giving out such loans, with websites when available. Remember that you may be able to qualify for a state loan based on your residency, your parents' residency, or the location of the school you're attending.

Alternative Loans

Alternative loans are loans that you, you and a co-borrower, or your parent can take out based on credit; usually the maximum you can borrow is for the cost of education minus all other financial aid received. Interest rates vary but are generally linked to the prime rate. Some of the many lenders who offer these types of loans are listed in the resources section at the end of this chapter. You can also ask your local bank for help or search the Internet for "alternative loans for students."

Questions to Ask Before You Take Out a Loan

In order to get the facts regarding the loan you're about to take out, ask the following questions:

1. What is the interest rate and how often is the interest capitalized? Your college's financial aid administrator (FAA) will be able to tell you this.

2. What fees will be charged? Government loans generally have an origination fee that goes to the federal government to help offset its costs, and a guarantee fee, which goes to a guaranty agency for insuring the loan. Both are deducted from the amount given to you.

3. Will I have to make any payments while still in school? It depends on the type of loan, but often you won't; depending on the type of loan, the government may even pay the interest for you while you're in school.

4. What is the grace period—the period after my schooling ends—during which no payment is required? Is the grace period long enough, realistically, for you to find a job and get on your feet? (A six-month grace period is common.)

5. When will my first payment be due and approximately how much will it be? You can get a good preview of the repayment process from the answer to this question.

6. Who exactly will hold my loan? To whom will I be sending payments? Who should I contact with questions or inform of changes in my situation? Your loan may be sold by the original lender to a secondary market institution, in which case you will be notified as to the contact information for your new lender.

7. Will I have the right to prepay the loan, without penalty, at any time? Some loan programs allow prepayment with no penalty but others do not.

8. Will deferments and forbearances be possible if I am temporarily unable to make payments? You need to find out how to apply for a deferment or forbearance if you need it.

9. Will the loan be canceled ("forgiven") if I become totally and permanently disabled, or if I die? This is always a good option to have on any loan you take out.

APPLYING FOR FINANCIAL AID

Now that you're aware of the types and sources of aid available, you will want to begin applying as soon as possible. You've heard about the Free Application for Federal Student Aid (FAFSA) many times in this chapter already, and should now have an idea of its importance. This is the form used by federal and state governments, as well as schools and private funding sources, to determine your eligibility for grants, scholarships, and loans. The easiest way to get a copy is to log onto www.ed.gov/offices/OSFAP/students, where you can find help in completing the FAFSA, and then submit the form electronically when you are finished. You can also get a copy by calling 1-800-4-FED-AID, or by stopping by your public library or your school's financial aid office. Be sure to get an original form, because photocopies of federal forms are not accepted.

The second step of the process is to create a financial aid calendar. Using any standard calendar, write in all of the application deadlines for each step of the financial aid process. This way, all vital information will be in one location, so you can see at a glance what needs to be done and when it's due. Start this calendar by writing in the date you requested your FAFSA. Then, mark down when you received it and when you sent in the completed form (or just the date you filled the form out online if you chose to complete the FAFSA electronically). Add important dates and deadlines for any other applications you need to complete for school-based or private aid as you progress though the financial aid process. Using and maintaining a calendar will help the entire financial aid process run more smoothly and give you peace of mind that the important dates are not forgotten.

Getting Your Forms Filed

Follow these three simple steps if you are not completing and submitting the FAFSA online:

1. Get an original Free Application for Federal Student Aid (FAFSA). Remember to pick up an original copy of this form, as photocopies are not accepted.

2. Fill out the entire FAFSA as completely as possible. Make an appointment with a financial aid counselor if you need help. Read the forms completely, and don't skip any relevant portions or forget to sign the form (or forget to have your parents sign, if required).

3. Return the FAFSA long before the deadline date. Financial aid counselors warn that many students don't file the forms before the deadline and lose out on available aid. Don't be one of those students!

When to Apply

Apply for financial aid as soon as possible after January 1 of the year in which you want to enroll in school. For example, if you want to begin school in the fall of 2002, then you should apply for financial aid as soon as possible after January 1, 2002. It is easier to complete the FAFSA after you have completed your tax return, so you may want to consider filing your taxes as early as possible as well. Do not sign, date, or send your application before January 1 of the year for which you are seeking aid. If you apply by mail, send your completed application in the envelope that came with the original application. The envelope is already addressed, and using it will make sure your application reaches the correct address.

Many students lose out on thousands of dollars in grants and loans because they file too late. Don't be one of them. Pay close attention to dates and deadlines.

After you mail in your completed FAFSA, your application will be processed in approximately four weeks. (If you file electronically, this time estimate is considerably shorter.) Then, you will receive a Student Aid Report (SAR) in the mail. The SAR will disclose your Expected Family Contribution (EFC), the number used to determine your eligibility for federal student aid.

Each school you list on the application may also receive your application information if the school is set up to receive it electronically.

You must reapply for financial aid every year. However, after your first year, you will receive a Student Aid Report (SAR) in the mail before the application deadline. If no corrections need to be made, you can just sign it and send it in.

Financial Need

Financial aid from many of the programs discussed in this chapter is awarded on the basis of need (the exceptions include unsubsidized Stafford, PLUS, consolidation loans, and some scholarships and grants). When you apply for federal student aid by completing the FAFSA, the information you report is used in a formula established by the United States Congress. The formula determines your Expected Family Contribution (EFC), an amount you and your family are expected to contribute toward your education. If your EFC is below a certain amount, you will be eligible for a Pell Grant, assuming you meet all other eligibility requirements.

There is no maximum EFC that defines eligibility for the other financial aid options. Instead, your EFC is used in an equation to determine your financial needs. Eligibility is a very complicated matter, but it can be simplified to the following equation: your contribution + your parents' contribution = expected family contribution (EFC). Student expense budget/cost of attendance (COA) minus EFC = your financial need.

The need analysis service or federal processor looks at the following if you are a dependent student:

- ▶ Family assets, including savings, stocks and bonds, real estate investments, business/farm ownership, and trusts
- ▶ Parents' ages and need for retirement income
- ▶ Number of children and other dependents in the family household
- ▶ Number of family members in college
- ▶ Cost of attendance, also called student expense budget; includes tuition and fees, books and supplies, room and board (living with parents, on

campus, or off campus), transportation, personal expenses, and special expenses such as childcare

A financial aid administrator calculates your cost of attendance and subtracts the amount you and your family are expected to contribute toward that cost. If there's anything left over, you're considered to have financial need.

Are You Considered Dependent or Independent?

Federal policy uses strict and specific criteria to make this designation, and that criteria applies to all applicants for federal student aid equally. A dependent student is expected to have parental contribution to school expenses, and an independent student is not.

You are an independent student if at least one of the following applies to you:

▶ You were born before January 1, 1979 (for the 2002–2003 school year).
▶ You are married (even if you're separated).
▶ You have legal dependents other than a spouse who get more than half of their support from you and will continue to get that support during the award year.
▶ You are an orphan or ward of the court (or were a ward of the court until age 18).
▶ You are a graduate or professional student.
▶ You are a veteran of the U.S. Armed Forces—formerly engaged in active service in the U.S. Army, Navy, Air Force, Marines, or Coast Guard or as a cadet or midshipman at one of the service academies—released under a condition other than dishonorable. (ROTC students, members of the National Guard, and most reservists are not considered veterans, nor are cadets and midshipmen still enrolled in one of the military service academies.)

If you live with your parents, and if they claimed you as a dependent on their last tax return, then your need will be based on your parents' income. You do not qualify for independent status just because your parents have decided to not claim you as an exemption on their tax return (this used to be the case but is no longer) or do not want to provide financial support for your college education.

Students are classified as dependent or independent because federal student aid programs are based on the idea that students (and their parents or spouse, if applicable) have the primary responsibility for paying for their postsecondary education. If your family situation is unusually complex and you believe it affects your dependency status, speak to a financial aid counselor at the school you plan to attend as soon as possible. In extremely limited circumstances a financial aid office can make a professional judgment to change a student's dependency status, but this requires a great deal of documentation from the student and is not done on a regular basis. The financial aid office's decision on dependency status is *final* and cannot be appealed to the U.S. Department of Education.

Gathering Financial Records

Your financial need for most grants and loans depends on your financial situation. Now that you've determined if you are considered a dependent or independent student, you will know whose financial records you need to gather for this step of the process. If you are a dependent student, then you must gather not only your own financial records, but also those of your parents because you must report their income and assets as well as your own when you complete the FAFSA. If you are an independent student, then you need to gather only your own financial records (and those of your spouse if you're married). Gather your tax records from the year prior to the one in which you are applying. For example, if you apply for the fall of 2003, you will use your tax records from 2002.

Filling Out the FAFSA

To help you fill out the FAFSA, gather the following documents:

- United States Income Tax Returns (IRS Form 1040, 1040A, or 1040EZ) for the year that just ended and W-2 and 1099 forms

- records of untaxed income, such as Social Security benefits, AFDC or ADC, child support, welfare, pensions, military subsistence allowances, and veterans' benefits
- current bank statements and mortgage information
- medical and dental expenses for the past year that weren't covered by health insurance
- business and/or farm records
- records of investments such as stocks, bonds, and mutual funds, as well as bank Certificates of Deposit (CDs) and recent statements from money market accounts
- Social Security number(s)

Even if you do not complete your federal income tax return until March or April, you should not wait to file your FAFSA until your tax returns are filed with the IRS. Instead, use estimated income information and submit the FAFSA, as noted earlier, just as soon as possible after January 1. Be as accurate as possible, knowing that you can correct estimates later.

MAXIMIZING YOUR ELIGIBILITY FOR LOANS AND SCHOLARSHIPS

Loans and scholarships are often awarded based on an individual's eligibility. Depending on the type of loan or scholarship you pursue, the eligibility requirements will be different. EStudentLoan.com (www.estudentloan.com/workshop.asp) offers the following tips and strategies for improving your eligibility when applying for loans and/or scholarships:

1. Save money in the parent's name, not the student's name.
2. Pay off consumer debt, such as credit card and auto loan balances.
3. Parents considering going back to school should do so at the same time as their children. Often, the more family members in school simultaneously, the more aid will be available to each.
4. Spend student assets and income first, before other assets and income.
5. If you believe that your family's financial circumstances are unusual, make an appointment with the financial aid administrator at your

school to review your case. Sometimes the school will be able to adjust your financial aid package to compensate.

6. Minimize capital gains.
7. Do not withdraw money from your retirement fund to pay for school. If you must use this money, borrow from your retirement fund.
8. Minimize educational debt.
9. Ask grandparents to wait until the grandchild graduates before giving them money to help with their education.
10. Trust funds are generally ineffective at sheltering money from the need analysis process, and can backfire on you.
11. If you have a second home, and you need a home equity loan, take the equity loan on the second home and pay off the mortgage on the primary home.

GENERAL GUIDELINES FOR LOANS

Before you commit yourself to any loans, be sure to keep in mind that they need to be repaid. Estimate realistically how much you will earn when you leave school, remembering that you will have other monthly obligations such as housing, food, and transportation expenses.

Once You Are in School

Once you have your loan (or loans) and you're attending classes, don't forget about the responsibility of your loan. Keep a file of information on your loan that includes copies of all your loan documents and related correspondence, along with a record of all your payments. Open and read all your mail about your education loan(s).

Remember also that you are obligated by law to notify both your financial aid administrator (FAA) and the holder or servicer of your loan if there is a change in your:

▶ name
▶ address

▶ enrollment status (dropping to less than half-time means that you will have to begin payment six months later)
▶ anticipated graduation date

After You Leave School

After graduation, you must begin repaying your student loan immediately, or begin after a grace period. For example, if you have a Stafford Loan you will be provided with a six-month grace period before your first payment is due; other types of loans have grace periods as well. If you haven't been out in the working world before, your loan repayment begins your credit history. If you make payments on time, you will build up a good credit rating, and credit will be easier for you to obtain for other things. Get off to a good start, so you don't run the risk of going into default. If you default (or refuse to pay back your loan) any number of the following things could happen to you as a result. You may:

▶ have trouble getting any kind of credit in the future.
▶ no longer qualify for federal or state educational financial aid.
▶ have holds placed on your college records.
▶ have your wages garnished.
▶ have future federal income tax refunds taken.
▶ have your assets seized.

To avoid the negative consequences of going into default in your loan, be sure to do the following:

▶ Open and read all mail you receive about your education loans immediately.
▶ Make scheduled payments on time; since interest is calculated daily, delays can be costly.
▶ Contact your servicer immediately if you can't make payments on time; he or she may be able to get you into a graduated or income-sensitive/income contingent repayment plan or work with you to arrange a deferment or forbearance.

There are a few circumstances under which you won't have to repay your loan. If you become permanently and totally disabled, you probably will not have to (providing the disability did not exist prior to your obtaining the aid) repay your loan. Likewise, if you die, if your school closes permanently in the middle of the term, or if you are erroneously certified for aid by the financial aid office you will probably also not have to repay your loan. However, if you're simply disappointed in your program of study or don't get the job you wanted after graduation, you are not relieved of your obligation.

LOAN REPAYMENT

When it comes time to repay your loan, you will make payments to your original lender, to a secondary market institution to which your lender has sold your loan, or to a loan servicing specialist acting as its agent to collect payments. At the beginning of the process, try to choose the lender who offers you the best benefits (for example, a lender who lets you pay electronically, offers lower interest rates to those who consistently pay on time, or who has a toll-free number to call 24 hours a day, 7 days a week). Ask the financial aid administrator at your college to direct you to such lenders.

Be sure to check out your repayment options before borrowing. Lenders are required to offer repayment plans that will make it easier to pay back your loans. Your repayment options may include:

▶ *Standard repayment*: full principal and interest payments due each month throughout your loan term. You will pay the least amount of interest using the standard repayment plan, but your monthly payments may seem high when you're just out of school.
▶ *Graduated repayment*: interest-only or partial interest monthly payments due early in repayment. Payment amounts increase thereafter. Some lenders offer interest-only or partial interest repayment options, which provide the lowest initial monthly payments available.
▶ *Income-based repayment*: monthly payments are based on a percentage of your monthly income.
▶ *Consolidation loan*: allows the borrower to consolidate several types of federal student loans with various repayment schedules into one loan.

This loan is designed to help student or parent borrowers simplify their loan repayments. The interest rate on a consolidation loan may be lower than what you're currently paying on one or more of your loans. The phone number for loan consolidation at the William D. Ford Direct Loan Program is 800-557-7392. Financial aid administrators recommend that you do not consolidate a Perkins Loan with any other loans since the interest on a Perkins Loan is already the lowest available. Loan consolidation is not available from all lenders.

▶ *Prepayment*: paying more than is required on your loan each month or in a lump sum is allowed for all federally sponsored loans at any time during the life of the loan without penalty. Prepayment will reduce the total cost of your loan.

It's quite possible—in fact likely—that while you're still in school your FFELP (Federal Family Education Loan Program) loan will be sold to a secondary market institution such as Sallie Mae. You will be notified of the sale by letter, and you need not worry if this happens—your loan terms and conditions will remain exactly the same or they may even improve. Indeed, the sale may give you repayment options and benefits that you would not have had otherwise. Your payments after you finish school, and your requests for information should be directed to the new loan holder.

If you receive any interest-bearing student loans, you will have to attend exit counseling after graduation, where the loan lenders or financial aid office personnel will tell you the total amount of debt and work out a payment schedule with you to determine the amount and dates of repayment. Many loans do not become due until at least six to nine months after you graduate, giving you a grace period. For example, you do not have to begin payment on the Perkins Loan until nine months after you graduate. This grace period is to give you time to find a good job and start earning money. However, during this time, you may have to pay the interest on your loan.

If for some reason you remain unemployed when your payments become due, you may receive an unemployment deferment for a certain length of time. For many loans, you will have a maximum repayment period of ten years (excluding periods of deferment and forbearance).

THE MOST FREQUENTLY ASKED QUESTIONS ABOUT FINANCIAL AID

Here are answers to some of the most frequently asked questions about student financial aid:

1. *I probably don't qualify for aid—should I apply for it anyway?*
   Yes. Many students and families mistakenly think they don't qualify for aid and fail to apply. Remember that there are some sources of aid that are not based on need. The FAFSA form is free—there's no good reason for not applying.

2. *Do I have to be a U.S. citizen to qualify for financial aid?*
   Students (and parents, for PLUS Loans) must be U.S. citizens or eligible noncitizens to receive federal and state financial aid. Eligible noncitizens are U.S. nationals or U.S. permanent nonresidents (with "green cards"), as well as nonresidents in certain special categories. If you don't know whether you qualify, speak to a financial aid counselor as soon as possible.

3. *Do I have to register with the Selective Service before I can receive financial aid?*
   Male students who are U.S. citizens or eligible noncitizens must register with the Selective Service by the appropriate deadline in order to receive federal financial aid. Call the Selective Service at 847-688-6888 if you have questions about registration.

4. *Do I need to be admitted at a particular university before I can apply for financial aid?*
   No. You can apply for financial aid any time after January 1. However, to get the funds, you must be admitted and enrolled in school.

5. *Do I have to reapply for financial aid every year?*
   Yes, and if your financial circumstances change, you may get either more or less aid. After your first year you will receive a Renewal Application which contains preprinted information from the previous year's FAFSA. Renewal of your aid also depends on your making satisfactory progress toward a degree and achieving a minimum GPA.

6. *Are my parents responsible for my educational loans?*

   No. You and you alone are responsible, unless they endorse or co-sign your loan. Parents are, however, responsible for federal PLUS Loans. If your parents (or grandparents or uncle or distant cousins) want to help pay off your loan, you can have your billing statements sent to their address.

7. *If I take a leave of absence from school, do I have to start repaying my loans?*

   Not immediately, but you will after the grace period. Generally, though, if you use your grace period up during your leave, you will have to begin repayment immediately after graduation, unless you apply for an extension of the grace period before it's used up.

8. *If I get assistance from another source, should I report it to the student financial aid office?*

   Yes—and, unfortunately, your aid amount will possibly be lowered accordingly. But you will get into trouble later on if you don't report it.

9. *Are federal work-study earnings taxable?*

   Yes, you must pay federal and state income tax, although you may be exempt from FICA taxes if you are enrolled full time and work less than 20 hours a week.

10. *My parents are separated or divorced. Which parent is responsible for filling out the FAFSA?*

    If your parents are separated or divorced, the custodial parent is responsible for filling out the FAFSA. The custodial parent is the parent with whom you lived the most during the past 12 months. Note that this is not necessarily the same as the parent who has legal custody. The question of which parent must fill out the FAFSA becomes complicated in many situations, so you should take your particular circumstance to the student financial aid office for help.

Financial Aid Checklist

____ Explore your options as soon as possible once you've decided to begin a training program.

____ Find out what your school requires and what financial aid they offer.

____ Complete and mail the FAFSA as soon as possible after January 1.

____ Complete and mail other applications by the deadlines.

____ Return all requested documentation promptly to your financial aid office.

____ Carefully read all letters and notices from the school, the federal student aid processor, the need analysis service, and private scholarship organizations. Note whether financial aid will be sent before or after you are notified about admission, and how exactly you will receive the money.

____ Gather loan application information and forms from your school or college financial aid office. You must forward the completed loan application to your financial aid office. Don't forget to sign the loan application.

____ Report any changes in your financial resources or expenses to your financial aid office so they can adjust your award accordingly.

____ Re-apply each year.

Financial Aid Acronyms Key

COA	Cost of Attendance (also known as COE, Cost of Education)
CWS	College Work-Study
EFC	Expected Family Contribution
EFT	Electronic Funds Transfer
ESAR	Electronic Student Aid Report
ETS	Educational Testing Service
FAA	Financial Aid Administrator
FAF	Financial Aid Form
FAFSA	Free Application for Federal Student Aid
FAO	Financial Aid Office/Financial Aid Officer
FDSLP	Federal Direct Student Loan Program
FFELP	Federal Family Education Loan Program
FSEOG	Federal Supplemental Educational Opportunity Grant
FWS	Federal Work-Study

PC	Parent Contribution
PLUS	Parent Loan for Undergraduate Students
SAP	Satisfactory Academic Progress
SC	Student Contribution
USED	U.S. Department of Education

FINANCIAL AID TERMS—CLEARLY DEFINED

accrued interest—interest that accumulates on the unpaid principal balance of your loan

capitalization of interest—addition of accrued interest to the principal balance of your loan that increases both your total debt and monthly payments

default—failure to repay your education loan

deferment—a period when a borrower, who meets certain criteria, may suspend loan payments

delinquency—failure to make payments when due

disbursement—loan funds issued by the lender

forbearance—temporary adjustment to repayment schedule for cases of financial hardship

grace period—specified period of time after you graduate or leave school during which you need not make payments

holder—the institution that currently owns your loan

in-school grace, and **deferment interest subsidy**—interest the federal government pays for borrowers on some loans while the borrower is in school, during authorized deferments, and during grace periods

interest-only payment—a payment that covers only interest owed on the loan and none of the principal balance

interest—cost you pay to borrow money

lender (originator)—puts up the money when you take out a loan; most lenders are financial institutions, but some state agencies and schools make loans too

origination fee—fee, deducted from the principal, which is paid to the federal government to offset its cost of the subsidy to borrowers under certain loan programs

principal—amount you borrow, which may increase as a result of capitalization of interest, and the amount on which you pay interest

promissory note—contract between you and the lender that includes all the terms and conditions under which you promise to repay your loan

secondary markets—institutions that buy student loans from originating lenders, thus providing lenders with funds to make new loans

servicer—organization that administers and collects your loan; may be either the holder of your loan or an agent acting on behalf of the holder

subsidized Stafford Loans—loans based on financial need; the government pays the interest on a subsidized Stafford Loan for borrowers while they are in school and during specified deferment periods

unsubsidized Stafford Loans—loans available to borrowers, regardless of family income; unsubsidized Stafford Loan borrowers are responsible for the interest during in-school, deferment periods, and repayment

FINANCIAL AID RESOURCES

In addition to the sources listed throughout this chapter, these are additional resources that may be used to obtain more information about financial aid.

Telephone Numbers

Federal Student Aid Information Center (U. S. Department of Education)

Hotline	800-4-FED-AID
	(800-433-3243)
TDD Number for Hearing-Impaired	800-730-8913
For suspicion of fraud or abuse of federal aid	800-MIS-USED
	(800-647-8733)
Selective Service	847-688-6888
Immigration and Naturalization (INS)	415-705-4205
Internal Revenue Service (IRS)	800-829-1040
Social Security Administration	800-772-1213
National Merit Scholarship Corporation	708-866-5100

Sallie Mae's college AnswerSM Service	800-222-7183
Career College Association	202-336-6828
ACT: American College Testing program (about forms submitted to the need analysis servicer)	916-361-0656
College Scholarship Service (CSS)	609-771-7725
TDD	609-883-7051
Need Access/Need Analysis Service	800-282-1550
FAFSA on the Web Processing/Software Problems	800-801-0576

Websites

www.ed.gov/prog_info/SFAStudentGuide
The Student Guide is a free informative brochure about financial aid and is available on-line at the Department of Education's Web address listed here.

www.ed.gov/prog_info/SFA/FAFSA
This site offers students help in completing the FAFSA.

www.ed.gov/offices/OPE/t4_codes
This site offers a list of Title IV school codes that you may need to complete the FAFSA.

www.ed.gov/offices/OPE/express
This site enables you to fill out and submit the FAFSA on line. You will need to print out, sign, and send in the release and signature pages.

www.career.org
This is the website of the Career College Association (CCA). It offers a limited number of scholarships for attendance at private proprietary schools. You can also contact CCA at 750 First Street, NE, Suite 900, Washington, DC 20002-4242.

www.salliemae.com
This is the website for Sallie Mae that contains information about loan programs.

www.teri.org
This is the website of The Educational Resource Institute (TERI), which offers alternative loans to students and parents.

www.nelliemae.com
This is the website for Nellie Mae; it contains information about alternative loans as well as federal loans for students and parents.

www.key.com
This is Key Bank's website, which has information on alternative loans for parents and students.

www.educaid.com
This is the website for Educaid, which offers both federal and alternative loans to students and parents.

Software Programs

Cash for Class
Redheads Software, Inc.
3334 East Coast Highway #216
Corona del Mar, CA 92625
Tel: 800-205-9581
Fax: 714-673-9039

Peterson's Award Search
Peterson's
P.O. Box 2123
Princeton, NJ 08543-2123
Tel: 800-338-3282 or 609-243-9111
www.petersons.com

Pinnacle Peak Solutions

(Scholarships 101)

Pinnacle Peak Solutions

7735 East Windrose Drive

Scottsdale, AZ 85260

Tel: 800-762-7101 or 602-951-9377

Fax: 602-948-7603

www.scholarships101.com

TP Software—Student Financial Aid

Search Software

TP Software

P.O. Box 532

Bonita, CA 91908-0532

Tel: 800-791-7791 or 619-496-8673

www.tpsoftware.com

Books and Pamphlets

The Student Guide
Published by the U.S. Department of Education, this is the handbook about federal aid programs. To get a printed copy, call 1-800-4-FED-AID.

Looking for Student Aid
Published by the U.S. Department of Education, this is an overview of sources of information about financial aid. To get a printed copy, call 1-800-4-FED-AID.

How Can I Receive Financial Aid for College?
Published from the Parent Brochures ACCESS ERIC website. Order a printed copy by calling 800-LET-ERIC or write to ACCESS ERIC, Research Blvd-MS 5F, Rockville, MD 20850-3172.

Cassidy, David J. *The Scholarship Book 2002: The Complete Guide to Private-Sector Scholarships, Fellowships, Grants, and Loans for the Undergraduate.* (Englewood Cliffs, NJ: Prentice Hall, 2001).

Chany, Kalman A. and Geoff Martz. *Student Advantage Guide to Paying for College 1997 Edition.* (New York: Random House, The Princeton Review, 1997.)

College Costs & Financial Aid Handbook, 18th ed. (New York: The College Entrance Examination Board, 1998).

Davis, Kristen. *Financing College: How to Use Savings, Financial Aid, Scholarships, and Loans to Afford the School of Your Choice* (Washington, DC: Random House, 1996).

Hern, Davis and Joyce Lain Kennedy. *College Financial Aid for Dummies* (Foster City, CA: IDG, 1999).

Peterson's Scholarships, Grants and Prizes 2002 (Princeton, NJ: Peterson's, 2001).

Ragins, Marianne. *Winning Scholarships for College: An Insider's Guide* (New York: Henry Holt & Company, 1994).

Scholarships, Grants & Prizes: Guide to College Financial Aid from Private Sources. (Princeton, NJ: Peterson's, 1998).

Schwartz, John. *College Scholarships and Financial Aid* (New York: Simon & Schuster, Macmillan, 1995).

Schlacter, Gail and R. David Weber. *Scholarships 2002* (New York: Kaplan, 2001).

Other Related Financial Aid Books

Annual Register of Grant Support (Chicago, IL: Marquis, annual).

A's and B's of Academic Scholarships (Alexandria, VA: Octameron, annual).

Chronicle Student Aid Annual (Moravia, NY: Chronicle Guidance, annual).

College Blue Book. Scholarships, Fellowships, Grants and Loans (New York: Macmillan, annual).

College Financial Aid Annual (New York: Prentice Hall, annual).

Directory of Financial Aids for Minorities (San Carlos, CA: Reference Service Press, biennial).

Directory of Financial Aids for Women (San Carlos, CA: Reference Service Press, biennial).

Financial Aids for Higher Education (Dubuque, IA: Wm. C. Brown, biennial).

Financial Aid for the Disabled and their Families (San Carlos, CA: Reference Service Press, biennial).

Leider, Robert and Ann. *Don't Miss Out: the Ambitious Student's Guide to Financial Aid* (Alexandria, VA: Octameron, annual).

Paying Less for College (Princeton, NJ: Peterson's, annual).

THE INSIDE TRACK

Who: Nicola Henri
What: Surgical Technician
Where: Bronx, NY

INSIDER'S STORY

I grew up in the Bronx, not too far away from where I work now. I spent my winters on the concrete sidewalks of New York. But every summer, because both my parents were teachers, I whiled away the hot months in the woods upstate where my family had a summer house on Lake George. It was a great opportunity for a kid to get out and experience nature. My neighbor up there, Mr. Lincoln, was the local veterinarian and my brother and I used to hang around his house and help him take care of the sick animals that were recuperating there. Well, one day a car hit a dog near the beach, and the dog's owner frantically brought the poor thing over to Dr. Lincoln's house. Dr. Lincoln had to perform emergency surgery if the dog was to survive, and he asked me if I would help him get everything ready because his assistant wasn't around. I did everything he told me, and stood by his side as he brought the dog, Duchess, back from the brink of the death. It was an amazing thing to witness. The atmosphere was tense, and I was seriously nervous, but it was like I was in a focused trance, and when it was all over—and we knew the dog was going to be all right—it was an incredible feeling. I was hooked and I didn't even know it at the time.

A few years later, my older sister Lucy, who is a nurse, told me about the actual occupation of surgical technician. Up until that point, I always thought that a nurse performed the technician's job; I didn't even know what a surgical technician was. I was really taken with the idea, so in the next few months I did some research and discussed the idea with my guidance counselor. We found a good program that was accredited by the AMA's Committee on Allied Health Education and Accreditation (CAHEA) in a community college nearby, and I was on my way.

The program was much harder than I expected. I had to study anatomy, physiology, microbiology; take classes on the care and safety of patients, use of anesthesia, and certain nursing procedures. I also learned how to sterilize instruments, prevent and control infection, and handle supplies, equipment, and special drugs. In addition to all that, I did supervised internships to gain exposure to a real surgical environment. But the work wasn't over when I graduated. I wanted to give myself the absolute best chance to find a well-paying job, so I decided to take the exam to get certified by the Liaison Council on Certification of Surgical Technologists. Studying for that exam was hard work, but once certified, I knew I was in position to score a good job, which I did almost immediately.

The job of a surgical technician is a vital one. You are an essential part of a team with an important mission: preserving the health of a human being. Knowing that you are a part of something that saved someone's life and prevented his or her loved ones from grief is unimaginably satisfying. But obviously, the outcome of surgery isn't always successful, and being able to deal with that reality is an important aspect of being a good technician. My confidence that the surgery team did the best they possibly could helps with that heartbreak, but it's still hard.

I would recommend becoming a surgical technician to anyone who is interested. It's not for the faint of heart, that's for sure. But if you are smart, love helping people, are a team player, and perform your best under stress, it could definitely be the job for you.

CHAPTER five

HOW TO LAND YOUR FIRST JOB

THIS CHAPTER EXPLAINS how to land your first job after you graduate from your training program. First you will learn who employs healthcare workers, and about their hiring processes. You will also learn how to conduct your job search using online resources, career placement services, hotlines, job fairs, and industry publications. Finally, there is an entire section devoted to the art of networking, which will help you now and throughout your career.

AS A GRADUATE of a healthcare training program, you will be in great demand for entry-level positions in your chosen field. Your mission is to learn about potential employers and decide the type of environment in which you want to work. Then, you need to use all the resources at your disposal to discover the job opportunities in your field. Just as you selected your career field and your training program, you can also select your first job. Even though you eventually will be chosen to fill a position out of a field of candidates by your new employer, you still have a lot of control over finding your first job.

The first step to gaining control over your job search is to understand who employs healthcare workers. With this information you can make a decision about the type of environment in which you want to work. The second step is to look into all the possibilities in your field. The more jobs you learn about the greater your choice. Devote as much time to your job search, and assume the same level of control as you did to the earlier phases of starting your career.

TYPES OF EMPLOYERS

For each healthcare position discussed in this book, there are many different types of employers. Each of these types of employer offers different benefits and challenges as a work environment. Some healthcare workers prefer the range of positions and opportunities for advancement offered at larger institutions. Other healthcare workers enjoy the benefits of working in a smaller practice where they may have a wider range of duties and can build relationships with their patients.

The most general employer is a hospital, which offers a multitude of positions for entry-level job seekers. Hospitals are designated as short-stay or long-term, depending on how much time a patient spends there before being discharged. The most common type of hospital is the *community* or *general hospital*, typically a small hospital where most people receive care.

A *teaching hospital* provides clinical training for medical students and other medical professionals and is usually part of a major medical school. *Public hospitals* are owned and operated by federal, state, or city governments, are usually located in the inner cities, and often treat patients who are unable to pay for services or who depend on Medicaid payments.

Another common type of employer is a *group medical practice.* In these, two or more doctors share a building or office, and each doctor may have a separate staff or they may share their staff. The doctors share the expenses of the building. These practices may include general practitioners or specialists such as optometrists and chiropractors. Group medical practices can range from large organizations to small offices with one or two assistants.

Health maintenance organizations (HMOs) are becoming an increasingly prevalent employer of healthcare workers. HMOs, like hospitals, employ a wide-range of healthcare workers. These group practices provide complete coverage for subscribers' health needs at a pre-established price. The patients (or their employers) pay a set amount each month; in turn, the HMO group provides care such as routine checkups at no extra charge, or at a very minimal charge. Members are usually locked into the plan for a specified period of time—often one year—and if the service they need is available within the HMO, they must use a selected HMO doctor.

Other employers of healthcare workers include *mental health facilities*, which provide medication, emotional support, and physical support to mentally ill patients. People employed by mental health facilities include mental health nursing assistants, medical records technicians, among others. *Hospices*, which provide support and care for terminally ill people in the final stage of their disease, help these patients live as comfortably and fully as possible. A hospice offers a program of services for both patients and their families so they can make the necessary preparations for death. A hospice may be a freestanding institution, a special wing at a hospital, or simply a few beds that can be made available to the program as needed.

Home healthcare provides nursing services in patients' homes. Patients may be any age and include those who expect to get better and resume work and daily activities as well as those who expect to die. Care may include everything from giving medication to providing physical therapy to housekeeping. Home health aides work in home healthcare.

Nursing homes provide long-term care for elderly patients. There are three types of nursing homes. A *residential care facility (RCF)* normally provides meals and housekeeping for the resident, plus some basic medical monitoring, and is geared toward residents who are fairly independent and do not need constant medical attention. An *intermediate care facility (ICF)* offers room and board and nursing care as necessary for those who can no longer live independently. A *skilled nursing facility (SNF)* provides round-the-clock nursing care plus physician coverage and is for patients who need intensive care plus services such as occupational therapy, physical therapy, and rehabilitation. Each of these facilities provides exercise and social programs as well. You will learn more about the rapidly growing field of eldercare in Chapter 8.

Surgicenters, also called outpatient centers, are ambulatory surgery centers equipped to perform routine surgical procedures that do not require an overnight stay. A surgicenter does not need the sophisticated and expensive equipment found in a hospital operating room. Minor surgeries, such as cosmetic surgery, abortions, tissue biopsies, hernia repair, cataract surgery, and some forms of cosmetic surgery, are typically performed in these facilities.

Surgical technologists, as well as medical records technicians and medical assistants, can find work at surgicenters.

Emergency clinics or *urgicenters* are usually run by private, for-profit organizations and provide up to 24-hour care on a drop-in basis. They offer quick help in an emergency when the nearest hospital is miles away, and they usually are open during the hours that most doctors' offices are closed. To minimize costs, they do not provide hospital beds. They deal with problems such as cuts that require sutures, sprains and bruises from accidents, and various infections.

TYPICAL HIRING PROCEDURES

Among most hospitals and physicians' centers, the hiring procedures are about the same. Applicants normally fill out an application for employment and participate in an interview. Many employers prefer that applicants fill out the application on site, so it is important to come prepared with all the necessary information. You should also bring along several copies of your resume, and submit one with your application. The human resources representative or employment recruiter may talk briefly with you when you turn in your application. Bringing everything with you will impress the employment recruiter.

For most positions, the employer will request that you take a drug test and a physical exam. They also will usually conduct a criminal background check and screen your references.

At certain hospitals and other institutions, you cannot apply for a position unless it is posted on the job board or applications have otherwise been requested. The job posting will most likely include a job description that outlines the duties of the position and the experience required. Job titles may vary at different institutions, but the duties involved will be similar. Here's a sample job posting for a medical assistant at a hospital:

Sample Job Description

Patient Care Technician

Job Summary: Provides direct patient care under the direction of a registered nurse or licensed practical nurse according to policy and procedure. Contributes to the safe and effective operation of the nursing unit. Provides direct patient care primarily for patients ages 12 and up.

Education: High school diploma or equivalent

Licensure: None

Experience: Previous exposure to training

Skills: Skills basic to completion of medical assistant course

Essential Physical and Mental Functions and Environmental Conditions: Able to see objects closely, as in reading, frequently. Able to see objects far away frequently. Able to discriminate color and perceive depth frequently.

Able to hear normal sounds with some background noise, as in answering telephone, frequently. Able to distinguish sounds, as in voice patterns, frequently.

Able to give and receive verbal communications continuously. Able to read and write written communications continuously.

Able to carry objects weighing 10 pounds or more frequently; able to carry objects weighing 49 pounds or less on occasion.

Able to sit 30 minutes consecutively, 1 hour per shift. Able to stand in place 10 minutes consecutively, 1 hour per shift. Able to remain on feet 4 hours consecutively, 7 hours per shift. Able to sustain awkward position 5 minutes consecutively, 2 hours per shift.

Able to perform motor skills such as bending, twisting, turning, kneeling, reaching out, reaching up, wrist turning, grasping, finger manipulation, feeling perception, fast response, frequently.

When a job title is unfamiliar, it is important to read the description. You may find that you are qualified for the job even though the title is not what you are used to.

Job openings are posted at hospitals for about five days, on average, and may be updated weekly. Many hospitals offer a job hotline number so prospective employees can keep up with the job openings. Smaller practices may take out ads in the newspapers or consult local hospitals for applicants.

The Application

If you have ever filled out an application for any kind of job, school, or financial aid before, the application for an entry-level position in healthcare will be similar. The application will ask for the following information:

▶ name, address, and Social Security number
▶ job information or previous work experience, including dates and reason for leaving
▶ skills or supervisory experience
▶ educational experience
▶ references, or you may be asked to sign a references release statement
▶ citizenship status

No question on the application should touch on a prospective employee's race, color, religion, national origin, age, sex, marital status, or disabilities. If there is such a question, you may leave it blank. The application should state that the company is an equal opportunity employer.

You will be asked to sign the application to verify that all the information is true and correct. The application will usually state that incorrect information is cause for immediate dismissal. Remember that most employers verify the information provided by applicants, so it is essential to be honest.

Your application will stay active on file at a hospital for six months. If you have not called to update it, it will be kept inactive for another six months. However, you may reapply or update your application at any time for other openings. In smaller healthcare practices, your application may or may not remain on file, depending on the size of the practice. Smaller practices usually do not have as high a turnover rate as hospitals, so there is little need to keep applications on file.

Employment Agencies

Employment agencies use the same hiring techniques as other companies. You will fill out an application, the agency will check your references, and, depending on the policy of the agency, you may have to take a drug test. The agency may or may not perform a criminal background check. You will find more information about finding work through an employment agency later in the chapter.

Federal and State Hiring Procedures

Federal and state institutions, such as public hospitals, must follow certain regulations when hiring employees. State regulations vary by state. These regulations are designed to make the hiring process fair for everyone, and are often followed by private institutions as well as public. Most hospitals hire according to federal and state hiring guidelines, but many small practices do not. A chiropractor from Chicago, Illinois, explains:

> I don't necessarily use federal or state guidelines for hiring, except the most commonly known, such as not discriminating. I have a very small business, and only one medical assistant is required to keep my office running smoothly. When I plan to hire someone for the front, I place an ad in the newspaper and accept applications from people for about a week, depending on whether I need someone immediately or not. I usually decide based on the applicant's experience and knowledge of handling patients. I can tell through an interview and a resume whether the applicant is right for the job.

Federal and state hiring procedures help larger companies keep certain criteria in mind as they hire large numbers of people. Employment requirements are much stricter in federal and state-owned and operated environments.

Examples of federal and state hiring procedures include:

► Companies must keep an application on active file for at least six months.
► Companies must clearly and adequately identify the requirements of a position in the vacancy announcement so that applicants understand the basis on which their application will be evaluated. This will also ensure that applicants possess the necessary skills to perform the work.

▶ Companies cannot set standards for any job that adversely affect the hiring chances of any one group of people, and the standards must be job-related, not person-related. *The Qualification Standards for General Schedule Positions*, or X-188, describes the legal standards of various jobs.

▶ Companies must interview at least three to five people for the opening.

▶ Companies cannot discriminate on the basis of race, religion, national origin, age, sex, marital status, or physical handicap.

▶ Any hiring tests must be related to the specific job for which the candidate has applied, and question responses cannot reduce the chances of minorities, women, or a disproportionate number of candidates in any single group.

CONDUCTING YOUR JOB SEARCH

Knowing the type of employer for which you want to work can make your job search much more focused. A focused candidate is always more appealing to an employer than a person who seems to be looking for just any job. However, it is important not to limit yourself too much. The more positions you apply for, the better your chances of landing a job. Major cities usually offer more employment opportunities than smaller towns, so be aware that your location has a lot to do with job availability. Also be aware that most job applicants apply for a number of openings before they find employment.

The keys to a successful job search are:

1. A clear idea of what you want.
2. An organized system for information related to your search.
3. A positive attitude.
4. Perseverance.

As a well-trained graduate of a healthcare program, you will have a pretty clear idea of what you want. You will learn more about keeping organized during your job search later in the chapter. A positive attitude will come from knowing what you want and knowing that you are thoroughly prepared for your new career, and this positive attitude will help you persevere if you do not meet with immediate success.

FINDING JOB OPPORTUNITIES

There are many methods for learning about job openings. The most successful is networking. Because networking is so important, there is a whole section devoted to networking later in the chapter. However, as you learned above, hospitals and other institutions rely on want ads, hotlines, and job boards for attracting qualified candidates. Here are some of the best methods for learning about job openings in today's healthcare market.

The Internet

The Internet can be a very efficient means of learning about job openings. It is especially useful if you are looking for jobs outside your local area. There are numerous sites on the web devoted to job postings and career development. These services are generally offered free to the user. Applicants can search in any geographic area in different job areas. Search results offer electronic job postings that are in many ways similar to traditional classified ads. One advantage of Internet postings is that employers are not usually as restricted in terms of space as they are in newspapers, so applicants will find more complete job descriptions and requirements.

In addition to finding job postings, these career sites also allow candidates to post their resumes on the site. To post your resume, you enter information in the searchable fields, such as job interests and qualifications. Employers can then search the sites' database for qualified candidates. If your qualifications match with an employer's search, your resume will be pulled up for the employer's consideration.

Some of the most popular general career sites on the web include:

6-Figure Jobs—www.6figurejobs.com
About.com—www.jobsearch.about.com/jobs/jobsearch
America's Employers—www.americasemployers.com
America's Job Bank—www.ajb.dni.us
Boston Herald's Job Find—www.jobfind.com
Career Builder—www.careerbuilder.com
Career.com—www.career.com

CareerNet—www.careers.org

CareerWeb—www.cweb.com

College Central Network—www.employercentral.com

Gary Will's Worksearch—www.garywill.com/worksearch

JobBank USA—www.jobbankusa.com

JobLynx—www.joblynx.com

JobSource—www.jobsource.com

Monster Board—www.monster.com

Occupational Outlook Handbook—www.stats.bls.gov

Salary.com—www.salary.com

Vault.com—www.vault.com

Wall Street Journal Careers—www.careers.wsj.com

Yahoo Careers—careers.yahoo.com

There are also sites devoted to healthcare that offer job postings, including

▶ www.healthgate.com
▶ www.medimorphus.com
▶ www.medsearch.com (the healthcare division of Monster.com)
▶ www.healthcareersonline.com
▶ www.hirehealth.com

These sites advertise jobs, allow you to post your resume, and in some cases offer career advice. In addition, many hospitals and companies also include job openings on their sites, For example, you can find out about job openings at the UCLA Medical Center at www.healthcare.ucla.edu and Reid Hospital and Healthcare Services in Richmond, Indiana, at www.reidhosp.com.

If you know the particular place you are interested in working, simply search for that name using any search engine, such as Yahoo! or Google. For more general searches, enter the term "hospital," "medical center," or "healthcare" and the city in which you are looking to find the websites of healthcare employers.

Career Services

As you learned in Chapter 3, one of the great advantages of a formal training program is the support offered to students when they launch their careers. Most vocational schools and colleges have a placement or career service center. Career services are offered to current students and recent graduates, and some schools offer ongoing career support for their graduates.

A career service center is one of your best resources. You can take advantage of career counseling, job boards, reference materials, resume writing assistance, and sometimes practice interviews. In addition, many employers recruit directly from technical or trade schools and colleges. This recruitment is often coordinated through the career service center. It is important to be connected with your career service center so you do not miss out on on-campus recruitment, such as interviews and job fairs.

Local and state employment services are another type of career service center. There are more than 2,700 such offices in the nation, and many employers automatically list their job openings at the local office. Whether you are looking for a job in private industry or with the state, these offices, which are affiliated with the federal employment service, are worth contacting.

Yet another type of career service center is private employment agencies. They will help you get a job if they think they can place you. Most employment agencies are paid by a company when they place a candidate with the company, so the agency will only send you for interviews with employers who they think will hire you. It is important to remember that the agency exists to serve the companies, not the job seeker, but it is the agency's interest to help you find a job.

In many cases, the agency staff will help you prepare a resume if you need one. Then they will contact employers they think might be interested in hiring you. Some may require a small registration fee whether or not you get a job through them. In general, these can be avoided and you should be extremely wary of any agency that charges substantial fees to help you find a job. With the bright prospects in the healthcare job market, you should have no trouble finding openings and getting your resume out there.

Classified Ads

The classified advertisements placed in newspapers, trade journals, and professional magazines are still a popular way to find qualified candidates. While these publications should not be the focus of your job search, they should not be overlooked entirely. The local newspaper might be a good source for finding a position at a small, local practice. Trade journals and professional magazines are not only a good place to find advertisements, but also a useful source of information on current medical trends.

When you find openings that interest you, follow up on each ad by the method requested. You may be asked to phone or send a resume. Record the date of your response, and if you don't hear from the employer within two or three weeks, place another call or send a polite note asking whether the job is still open.

Temporary Agencies

Temporary work is a good way to get a handle on the job market. Many agencies specialize in placing people in short-term healthcare jobs. Nurses, nursing aides, and medical technicians are among the types of workers most in demand. Temporary employment can increase your job skills, your knowledge of a particular field, and your chances of finding out about permanent positions. A temporary job can also give you a chance to test out different work environments. As a temporary medical assistant you might work in a small practice one week, and a large hospital another week.

To find temporary work, you can register with a temporary agency. The process is the same as for employment agencies. In fact, many employment agencies also function as temporary agencies. You may even work for the agency as a temporary while the agency is also working to place you in a permanent position. And in some cases, your temporary position can become permanent over time.

Job Fairs

As you learned earlier, most colleges and universities hold at least one job fair per year, usually coordinated through the career service center. Job fairs are not just for near-grads looking for employment; they also are useful for students who are interested in developing their networking skills. You should attend job fairs in business attire and bring along at least ten copies of your resume.

Job fairs are also held outside of the school setting. Large companies may also hold job fairs to hire employees. There are also job fairs for industries such as healthcare, which numerous employers attend to find candidates. These fairs are advertised in local newspapers and in industry publications.

Job Hotlines

Each city has its own job hotline monitored by the state employment agency. You can call your local state employment agency for the phone number of the hotline that offers daily lists of jobs in your area. For a list of 5,000 job hotline numbers, look for the *National Job Hotline Directory* in the reference department of your local library. Some hospitals and medical centers also have job hotlines.

STAYING ORGANIZED

One of the keys to a successful job search is organization. There is a lot of information to keep track of, and you need to develop a system that works for you. Any system of organization must include a calendar, a file system, and an address or contact list.

When you begin your search dedicate a desk or wall calendar to record your efforts. Use this calendar to keep track of all your activities including:

▶ date on which you applied for any opening whether by mail or in person
▶ date on which you contacted anyone regarding job opportunities
▶ dates of any upcoming job fairs

▶ dates on which you sent thank-you letters or any other related correspondence

▶ dates of any appointments for interviews

▶ dates of any follow-up calls—either to be returned or made

One of the most important functions of the calendar is to help you record your progress and to guide your next step. For example, if you see on your calendar that you applied for a position two weeks ago and have not yet heard from the employer, you will know that it is time to make a follow-up call. You can also see if you have not sent any resumes out for a week. This will remind you to aggressively pursue leads for new opportunities.

Develop a file system to keep all your papers in order. You might have one file for cover letters, filed in order by date; another file for all the job postings to which you have applied; another file for research you have conducted about specific employers; and so on. These files will be very useful and should be kept close at hand. For example, when you are in the midst of a busy job search it is often difficult to remember the names of all the people you have contacted regarding your search. Sometimes you will receive a phone call from someone whose name does not, at first, sound familiar. If you have a file of cover letters next to your phone you can quickly look through them to find the letter you sent to the person who is now calling you about a job opportunity.

Finally, you need an address book or Personal Digital Assistant (PDA) that has all the vital information for your important contacts. Your contact listing should also record how you know the person and the important dates regarding your communication. You will find more information about keeping track of contacts in the next section about networking.

NETWORKING

Networking is one of the best means of finding out about job openings. It is also a skill that you should rely on throughout your career to advance and to learn about important industry developments. Networking opens doors you never knew about and helps you find a job with the help of a reference, which is sometimes better than searching on your own. Many times employers will hire you based on the recommendation of a trusted source.

What Is Networking?

A network is a group of people who are connected to you personally, socially, and professionally. Or, a network is the people you know, plus the people they know, and so on. Networking means developing your network and calling on this network of people for advice and support. Networking is an extension of something that we all do everyday, and it should be an ongoing part of your career, not just something you rely on to help you find a job. Many people find the idea of networking intimidating, and, often, it is because they don't like to ask for help.

It is important to remember that a network is not a one-way proposition. When you develop your network, you are also making yourself available as a source of advice and support. A network is mutually beneficial and many people enjoy offering their advice. Networking can be as simple as asking your uncle for the name of his mechanic, or as extensive as contacting a wide range of people when you are looking for a new job.

You never know what opportunity someone will be able to find for you. Only about 20 to 30 percent of job vacancies are advertised; many employers look for employees by word-of-mouth. This is called the "hidden job market." In today's competitive climate, successful candidates must pursue all possible outlets. Networking is probably the most important.

Building Your Network

When you are building your network, consider all possible living, breathing human resources: family, friends (including neighbors and parents of classmates), school personnel (teachers, counselors, alumni, administrators), previous employment contacts (employers, coworkers, customers, competitors), professionals (doctors, dentists, practicing professionals in your field), and community (business people, members of clubs, associations, chambers of commerce, and religious groups).

You also can use magazine articles, newspapers, or other general publicity to begin targeting people you would like to include in your network. For example, if you read an article about a local doctor in the newspaper and she sounds like someone for whom you would like to work, you can include the doctor's name among the people you plan to contact.

It is important not to overlook any possibilities. However, you need to make contact with each person you plan to use in your network. For a job search, you will want to focus your network building efforts on those people who have connections to your field. However, you may have to do some networking to *find* those people. For example, you may not know about your cousin's wife who works as a nurse in your local hospital until you get in touch with your aunt.

Make a list of your core contacts. These will be the people you rely on in everyday life—your friends, family, and community leaders. Even if these people do not work directly in your field they may know other people who do. Your core contacts can put you in touch with other people who may be helpful.

Next list everyone you know in the healthcare field. This will include the contacts you have developed at school and through any work experience you gained as a student. You can also include the healthcare professionals who have cared for you. For example, if you have a regular doctor, you can include him or her in your network.

Making Contact

It's time to begin asking others for help. Contacting a whole list of people for favors can seem like a nerve-wracking prospect. However, the key to successful networking lies in understanding that you aren't asking for a giant favor that puts you in debt to others. You are subtly empowering the other party while not asking for much in return.

When you contact someone—whether by phone, e-mail, or letter—first identify yourself clearly. If someone referred you to this person, identify not only yourself but your referral source as well. Then briefly explain why you are contacting the person. If you are contacting the person by phone, make sure it is clear that you are not asking for the person's help on the spot. Give the person an opportunity to set up an appointment to talk to you at greater length at another time.

In a letter or e-mail you can explain your objective in more detail, but you should still be fairly brief. Your initial contact should serve to introduce yourself, if you do not already know the person, and to state your objective in contacting the person. Most likely you will then make an appointment to talk to the person further if the contact thinks he or she can be of help to you.

Your contacts' willingness to help you will depend largely on how your requests are phrased. Keep your requests for help brief, conversational, and low-key. Be sincere.

- Ask contacts if it is a good time to talk for about 10 minutes, and, if they have the time, then explain your job goals and ask them if they have any information to share with you.
- Explain that you don't expect an immediate answer, and ask if you can call them back or meet on a specific date.
- Use phrases such as "Would it be possible to make an appointment to get your thoughts about my job search?" or "Would you have some time to talk to me about getting started in your field?"

Keep it light and pleasant. If you are nervous, recite what you plan to say before you make that important call.

Last, but certainly not least, thank your contacts for their time after your initial contact. It is essential to thank any contacts that you meet with and who give you their time and advice. Write a letter immediately to let them know you really appreciate their help and that you are grateful for their willingness to mention you to their colleagues. Thank them as well for any referrals they may have given you. Also let them know that you will keep them posted about what happens. Many contacts will be interested to know that their input has helped you.

Expanding Your Contacts

Ask the people you contact for other referrals. Your contacts may call the referrals to prepare them for your call and to introduce you and your objective before you call.

Don't be afraid to contact people directly, even if they are complete strangers. You are paying them a compliment by contacting them. People like to talk about themselves. And remember, everybody likes a good listener. You are empowering these people when you ask for their personal advice, information, and wisdom.

Making the Most of Your Contacts

The contacts that you establish in your field can helpful to you in many ways in your job search and throughout your career. One of the most important things you can do to make good use of your contacts is being prepared. You should prepare in the same way you would for an interview.

If you do not know the person, find out what you can about him or her before the appointment. You may be able to learn about the person from your original contact. If the person works in your field, find out about the place where he or she work. The better informed you are the more pertinent and intelligent questions you can ask.

This is your second task: come to the interview prepared with a list of questions. Remember, you asked for the interview so it is your responsibility to guide the conversation. Do not expect someone to simply tell you all they know without any prompting. Having a well thought out list of questions will demonstrate your respect for your contact's time as well as your organization and focus. You can ask questions not only about job prospects but also about the field in general and the person's career advice.

Organizing Your Contact List

You will need to keep track of your contacts. Keep all your contact names and their information in one place. You can use index cards, a notebook, a PDA, or a computer database. Use any tracking system that is comfortable for you. Set up your network file to include the following contact information:

- ▶ name of contact
- ▶ address and telephone number
- ▶ how you met this person
- ▶ occupation
- ▶ date last contacted
- ▶ conversation summary
- ▶ names of referrals
- ▶ date of thank-you letter
- ▶ other comments

Maintaining Your Network

Keep in touch. Check in with your contacts every month to let them know how your job hunt is progressing. Keeping visible will generate further job leads. The key to faster success in your networking efforts is follow-up.

Even though the majority of follow-up calls will not produce valuable new information or insights, a timely call can jog your contact's memory and get results. In addition to writing thank-you notes, you can clip and send relevant articles or follow up on personal information shared in your conversation. Perhaps your contact mentioned a favorite sports team or a type of music they like; if you mention this again, you are likely to stand out in his or her memory.

PUTTING IT ALL TOGETHER

Make use of all the methods described above to find job opportunities. Devote the most time to the most effective methods. Networking is generally considered to the most effective job search method so dedicate a good portion of your effort to building and tapping into your network. Classified ads are considered the least effective job search method so allot the least amount of your time to combing help wanted ads.

However, there are some exceptions in the case of healthcare careers. For example, hospitals, especially public hospitals, must post opening and interview a certain number of candidates. So even if your uncle is the head of the hospital you will still have to go through the same process as all the other applicants.

Read on to discover how to turn a job opportunity into a job offer in the next chapter about resumes, cover letters, and interviews.

THE INSIDE TRACK

Who: Don Olivera
What: Home Health Aide
Where: Phoenix, Arizona

INSIDER'S STORY

I started working as a home health aide three years ago. I was initially thinking of
becoming a nurse, but I didn't feel like I knew enough about the particulars of the work
to commit to the training that would be required to become an LPN. I found out that the
only training required to be a home health aide was a two-week training course
through the home care agency, and it seemed like a good way to get started working in
healthcare.

When I started working in home care, I would see two or three clients a day, mostly
people who were fairly self-sufficient but needed help with everyday tasks like bathing
or getting dressed, or needed help around the house with laundry or preparing meals.
These were usually people who were temporarily disabled or recovering from an
accident or injury, so their care was pretty short-term. Recently, I've been doing more
long-term work with elderly people who need a lot of help at home but aren't ready to
(or just don't want to) enter a nursing home or assisted-living situation.

Although it can be tiring, I like my work a lot. It feels great to have a role in enabling
people to remain fairly independent and keep living in their own homes, where they
have often been living for 25 years or more. Most of the other aides I know are women,
and several of my older male clients have told me that it's actually nice for them to
have a male caretaker.

I plan to start my LPN training next fall. The program lasts about a year, and I'm
thinking about eventually going on to become an R.N. After I'm licensed, I'd like to stay
in the home care field, rather than working in a hospital or nursing home. I'm especially
looking forward to the pay increase that will come with being licensed—one of the
hardest things about working as a home care aide is that the pay is very low, and
there's not much potential for raises, so it can sometimes feel unrewarding financially.
The upside to that, of course, is knowing that I am an essential part of someone's daily
life, that they depend on me and appreciate the services I provide.

CHAPTER six

TURNING JOB OPPORTUNITIES INTO OFFERS

IN THE LAST CHAPTER you learned about the best methods you can use to find out about job opportunities. The real challenge is to take those opportunities and to turn them into offers. In this chapter you will learn how to write cover letters and resumes that will get you noticed. Then you will discover the secrets to making a great impression in an interview so that you get the job offer.

NOW THAT you have done the work to learn about job openings, you are ready to take the next step—applying for the position. For some health-care positions, as you have already learned, you apply for positions by filling out an application. Even when you can apply with an application, you will need to have a resume ready. Often you will be asked to submit your resume along with the completed application, or when you go for an interview.

For other positions—ones that you have learned about through networking, through the Internet, or in a classified ad, for example—you will most likely send a cover letter and your resume. Your cover letter and resume are your introduction to your potential employer and it is essential that they make a great first impression. Read on to learn how to write a cover letter and resume that will get you noticed, and get you to the next step—the interview.

WRITING YOUR COVER LETTER

The quality of your written correspondence is a critical part of what makes an employer interested in calling you for an interview. And your cover letter is what a potential employer will read first. In a profession like healthcare where accuracy and neatness can mean life or death, a messy or sloppy cover letter will certainly put an end to your candidacy for a job.

A cover letter, or query letter, is written to state your interest in obtaining a job with a company and to explain why you are the right candidate for the job. A good cover letter should be neat, clear, brief, and, most important, specific. It should be no more than two or three paragraphs long. Ideally, you should send this letter to the person who is making the hiring decision, or the person selecting candidates for interviews. If you don't know that person's name, call the company and ask to whom you should write. Sometimes, the company will not make this information available, and in this case you can address your letter to "human resources manager" or "human resources department."

Begin your letter by explaining why you are writing. Let the person know that you are interested in being considered for the job, and how you learned about the opening. You can also write to a large company, for example a big hospital, to inquire about openings and express your interest in being considered. However, it is generally much more effective to apply for a specific opening. If you learned about the opening through your networking efforts, be sure to mention the name of the person who is recommending you and what that person's connection is with the person to whom you are writing. For example, "I am interested in being considered for the medical assistant position in your office. Ray Thompson, who visits your office as a sales representative for PhisoMed, informed me that you are currently seeking to fill an opening." If you learned of the position through the Internet, the newspaper, or another source you should state this.

Next, you should express why you are specifically interested in or qualified for this position. It is important to be as specific as possible about the position for which you are applying. Do some research about the hospital or medical practice and incorporate that information into your letter. Of course, it is important to be honest. Do not say that you have always been interested in working with infants if this is not true. If you cannot write an effective letter that convincingly and honestly states why you are interested in working at a particular medical practice, then perhaps this job is not right for you.

The second paragraph of your letter should explain in more detail about your qualifications and particular strengths. However, you cover letter is intended to introduce your resume not to replicate it. So, use your cover letter to highlight two or three points on your resume that are specifically related to the job for which you are applying. Your cover letter is also an opportunity to describe your personal qualities that are perhaps not explicitly stated in your resume. These statements are always more persuasive when you can offer tangible proof of your personal traits. For example, if you would like to convey that you are organized and accurate in your work, you might tie this quality to particular achievement.

Always close your letter by thanking the reader for his or her attention to your letter, and add that you look forward to hearing back soon. Before you send your cover letter proofread it very carefully. Double-check the spelling of the person's name and the name of the medical practice. If you can, have someone you know read the letter as well.

Use the following examples to help you draft a personalized cover letter.

135 Lariott Court
Tampa, FL 12345

June 23, 2002

Gary Johnson
Personnel Department
St. Joseph's Hospital
P.O. Box 1565
Clearwater, FL 12345

Dear Mr. Johnson:

I am writing to inquire about openings for medical assistants in your hospital. I have read and heard many favorable things about your hospital, and I feel that this would be the perfect work environment for me. The fact that St. Joseph's Hospital is a small but rapidly growing hospital presents interesting challenges and unique opportunities, and I am eager to be considered for a position as a medical assistant.

I am a 2001 graduate of the medical technology assistant program at Clearwater Community College and I am a certified medical assistant. Prior to attending school, I worked for five years as an executive assistant at a real estate office and I have excellent word processing and office management skills. As part of my program, I worked for a semester at Clearwater General Hospital. I was responsible for pulling patients' records for their clinic visits and on completion of my internship my supervising nurse, Karen Brown, commended me for my accurate and consistent work.

I am confident that my skills as a medical assistant would be an asset to the staff at St. Joseph's. Thank you for considering my inquiry. I have enclosed my resume for your reference, and I look forward to hearing from you.

Sincerely,

Emily J. Small

Emily J. Small
Enc: Resume

6895 Peabody Ave.
Dallas, TX 45768

July 2, 2002

Dr. Elizabeth Townsend
South Dallas Women's Health Clinic
123 Depot Street
Dallas, TX 45769

Dear Dr. Townsend:

I am writing on the recommendation of Dr. Mary Carlisle, who was my advisor at Bryman College. Dr. Carlisle informed me that there is currently an opening for a radiologic technologist at the Women's Health Clinic. I am a trained sonographer and I am particularly interested in working in obstetrics. I am aware of the Women's Health Clinic's reputation as Dallas's leading obstetrics practice and I am very interested in being considered for this position.

I earned my associate's degree from Bryman in December 2001 and I am certified by the American Registry of Diagnostic Medical Sonographers. I completed my clinical class work at South Dallas General Hospital. At South Dallas General, I found that I have a good rapport with patients, doctors, and other technicians. My clinic supervisor was particularly impressed with my ability to work efficiently while still putting patient care first.

I have enclosed my resume and Dr. Carlisle's letter of recommendation for your consideration. Thank you for your attention to my letter. I can be reached at 777-555-1323, at the address above, or by e-mail at janderson@email.com. I look forward to hearing from you.

Sincerely,

James T. Anderson

James T. Anderson
Enc: Resume

WRITING YOUR RESUME

The word *resume* originates from the French word *resumer*, which means "to summarize," and that is exactly what you will do with your resume. Your resume is a snapshot of your education, work experience, special abilities, and skills. This summary can act as your introduction by mail, your calling card if you are applying in person, and a convenient reference when you are filling out an application form or being interviewed. A resume is usually a required component of any job application.

The purpose of a resume is to capture the interest of potential employers so they will call you for a personal interview. To create a complete picture of yourself include the following sections:

▶ Objective
▶ Education
▶ Work experience and/or employment history
▶ Special skills or qualifications
▶ Related non-work experience

At the top of your resume, put your name, address, e-mail address, and phone number.

Objective

Under your name and address you should state your job objective. Describe briefly the type of job you hope to obtain. In your resume you should state your more general career goal. Your cover letter will give you the opportunity to talk specifically about a particular position for which you are applying. However, you can also tailor your resume for a specific position.

Educational Background

Your education will be very important to many healthcare employers as they will check your resume to make sure you have at least met the minimum training requirements for the position. If training is necessary for a position for which you are applying, you will want to list your education following your objective—especially if you have not yet accrued a great deal of work experience in your new field.

When listing your educational background, start with your most recent training and work backward. Employers want to know your highest qualifications at a glance. For each educational experience, include dates attended, name and location (city and state) of school, and degree or certificate earned. If you have advanced degrees (college and beyond), it is not necessary to include your high school education.

Work Experience

You may not have an established work history in healthcare, but your past work experience, summer jobs, part-time and volunteer work can be presented to highlight your skills and accomplishments in a way that will be pertinent to potential employers. For example if you were a manager at a restaurant, and you are now applying for a position as a medical assistant you can stress the organization skills required to manage the calendar, order supplies, and so on.

Special Skills

You may wish to include another section called "Skills," "Related experience," or "Personal qualifications." Write down any skills such as typing, knowledge of software programs, knowledge of office equipment, supervisory experience, and any other skill that directly applies to your future job.

Ways to Organize Your Resume

There are two main methods for organizing a resume. The different styles enable you to present your experience in the most advantageous manner.

The most common resume format is *chronological.* In this format you list your employment experience chronologically starting with your most recent job. For each job, list the name and location of the company for which you worked, the dates you were employed, and the position(s) you held. The order in which you present this information will depend on what you are trying to emphasize. For example, if you want to call attention to the type or level of job you held, you should put the job title first. But you must be consistent. Summer employment or part-time work should be identified as such, and you will need to specify the months in the dates of employment for positions you held for less than a year.

A chronological resume works well for a person with a regular job history, that is, with no major gaps in employment. But even if your work experience has been interrupted to complete your education, this should not prevent you from using the chronological format, as the dates that you attended school will be clearly stated. The advantages to the chronological resume are that it is easy to read, it is the format that many employers are used to, and it is straightforward.

On the other hand, the *functional* resume emphasizes what you *can* do rather than what you *have* done. It is useful for people who have an irregular work history or who have relevant skills that would not be properly highlighted in a chronological listing of jobs. The functional resume concentrates on your qualifications—anything from familiarity with hospital procedures to organizational skills or managerial experience. You can mention specific jobs, but they are not the primary focus of this type of resume. This type of resume is useful if you have limited work experience—or if your work experience is a different field.

There is also a third type of resume that combines the chronological and functional formats. A *combination* resume allows you to present your skills as well as a chronological list of jobs you have held. You get the best of both resumes. This format might work best if you have a significant work history in another field.

Sample Chronological Resume

JEAN THOMPSON
1234 Third Street
Kansas City, MO 64131
816-555-4510
JeanT@kansascitythompsons.com

OBJECTIVE
To obtain a position as a medical assistant in a private practice.

EDUCATION
Medical assistant certificate, May 2002
Kansas City Community College, 7910 Troost Ave., Kansas City, MO 64131
GPA: 3.95
Great Lions High School, Kansas City, MO 64130, June 1997
GPA: 3.2

WORK EXPERIENCE
Candy striper, nurse aide volunteer, 1999–2001
St. Mary's Hospital, Kansas City, MO 64130
• Served meals and helped patients eat, dress, and bathe.
• Delivered messages and answered patient call bells.
• Completed daily filing and answered telephones.
• Inventoried, stored, and moved supplies.

Evening manager, September 1996–May 2002
King Seafood Restaurant, Kansas City, MO 64133
• Arranged staff schedule and supervised staff of thirty.
• Responsible for all nightly receipts, including balancing register and making bank deposits.
• Monitored and ordered supplies.
• Coordinated with day manager to ensure smooth operations.
• Waited on tables and greeted customers.

COMPUTER EXPERIENCE
Typing 65 wpm
Macintosh, IBM, Claris Works, Microsoft Office Suite, WordPerfect, Lotus 1-2-3, e-mail

ACTIVITIES
Volunteer at Meltrice's Nursing Home in Wilmington, MO, and at local food shelters.

REFERENCES
References furnished by Kansas City Community College, Career Planning and Placement Office,
Griffin Hall, Kansas City, MO 64131; 816-555-1231

Sample Functional Resume

JACK WOODSON
1234 Second Ave.
Jackson, MS 10908
601-555-9876
jw@jackmail.com

OBJECTIVE

To obtain a position as a radiologic technologist.

VOLUNTEER NURSING ASSISTANT

Two years volunteer experience as nursing assistant in competitive hospital

Performed typical nursing assistant duties, including patient care in the pediatric ward

Measured patients' vital statistics using the latest technology

Became familiar with radiologic technology by taking bone X rays

CLINIC ASSISTANT

Assisted medical assistant with paperwork and filing

Ran errands and answered phones

EDUCATION

Associate degree in radiologic technology, June 2001

University of Mississippi Medical Center, Jackson, Mississippi

Major: Radiology

GPA: 3.8/4.0

COMPUTER SKILLS

Microsoft Office 2000

REFERENCES

References available upon request.

Sample Combination Resume

Jennifer Perkins

1234 Obart St.

Orlando, FL 33054

407-555-7656

jennifer_perkins@unc.edu

OBJECTIVE

To obtain a position as a physical therapy aide.

QUALIFICATIONS

Skilled, certified physical therapy aide with three years of experience as a nursing assistant. Specialized in geriatric physical therapy at University of North Carolina. Devoted to the health and well being of my patients with an especially strong rapport with aging patients.

EDUCATION

College of Allied Health

University of North Carolina, Chapel Hill, NC

Associate Degree in Physical Therapy, May 2002

Orlando Area Technical College

Nursing Assistant Certificate, December 1997

RELATED CLINICAL TRAINING

- Rehabilitation therapy for stroke patients. Semester-long clinic at Chapel Hill General Hospital.
- Water-based therapy course and clinic.
- Anatomy and physiology.

RELATED EXPERIENCE

Nursing assistant, St. Jude's Hospital, Geriatric ward, Orlando, Florida 1/98–12/00

- Served meals and assisted patients with eating.
- Bathed and dressed patients and made beds.
- Assisted patients with standing and walking.
- Took patients' vital signs and maintained records.
- Explained medication regimes to patients and family members.

RELATED SKILLS

Fluent in Spanish, proficient in Microsoft Office 2000.

REFERENCES

Available upon request.

COVER LETTER AND RESUME WRITING TIPS

Following are some basic guidelines to help you write a great cover letter and resume. There are entire books dedicated to this topic, the best of which you will find in the resources at the back of this book. However, this abbreviated list includes all the essential information.

- ▶ Present your information in an organized and consistent manner.
- ▶ Proofread. Not once but twice.
- ▶ Include ample white space on the page.
- ▶ Try to limit your resume to one page, but do not crowd it. Go to two pages if necessary.
- ▶ Qualify *how* you did a job rather than listing tasks.
- ▶ Quantify your accomplishments whenever possible.
- ▶ Use action verbs. Avoid the passive voice whenever possible.
- ▶ Be positive and confident, but don't lie or embellish.
- ▶ Use good quality paper in a subtle color. Use the same paper for your cover letter and resume.
- ▶ Use a good quality printer. Make sure the type is legible and even in tone.
- ▶ See Appendix B for more resume and cover letter resources.

ACING YOUR INTERVIEW

Now you are ready to tackle the most important part of your job search: the interview. Employers read cover letters and resumes to select candidates to interview, but the interview is the process through which they make hiring decisions. It is the employer's chance to meet candidates in person and ask them more in-depth questions. An interview is also an opportunity for a candidate to find out more about the position and the place of employment. Your chance of acing your interview happens before you even sit down to face your interviewer. Fortunately, this part—preparation—is totally within your control.

Preparing for Your Interview

Preparation will enable you to be confident, overcome interviewing inexperience, and sell yourself and your qualifications. When you go to your interview you will bring your resume and you should also bring a personal inventory. This personal inventory is what you will have created to help you answer possible interview questions. It is a description of your strengths and a list of examples and anecdotes that support the information on your resume.

One way to create a personal inventory is to write a short personal autobiography. Write down the details of your work and educational experiences. Be sure to include information about your motivations and goals. Think about any particular moments of which you are proud or that demonstrate your strengths. As you write your personal inventory, you can refer to your resume. Try to make sure you have more to say about each item on your resume. One common interview technique is to go through the candidate's resume and ask for more information about each experience. The exercise of creating your personal inventory will help prepare you to give thoughtful and useful answers to these questions.

Knowing more about yourself is only part of your task. You also need to research the company or organization to which you are applying so you feel more comfortable and can demonstrate genuine interest in the position during the interview. The Internet is a great source of information. If the company has its own website, you should have access to all the information you will need to prepare. If the company does not have its own website you might be able to find information about the company on other sites. The public library is another good source for this kind of information, as are health publications. The idea is to converse intelligently about the company during the interview, and to have enough information to ask knowledgeable questions.

Dress for success. What you wear says a lot about your personality and attitude. Dress in a way that shows you are proud of yourself and your accomplishments. For men, a conservative suit with a white shirt and contrasting tie, and well-shined shoes should be appropriate. For women, a jacket and skirt or dress in navy or black, neutral or sheer hose, simple pumps, and simple makeup are appropriate for most situations. It is generally better to err on the conservative side when making decisions about dressing for an interview.

Allow plenty of time for the interview. It is possible that you may interview with more than one person during the interview cycle. You won't be at your best if you are worried about another appointment. If you are scheduling more than one interview a day allow more time than you think you will need between interviews. This will allow you to approach each interview in a calm and unhurried manner.

Arrive at the interview site ten minutes before the interview. Punctuality shows your respect for the interviewer, and your professionalism. Allow extra travel time so you can find the employer's location and accommodate any unexpected transportation trouble, such as heavy traffic.

Keep yourself in a positive frame of mind. Remember that you are there to discuss job-related topics. Keep in mind the personal inventory you created; focus on your strengths and the positive stories you have prepared. Also remember that the interviewer is looking for a new employee. Most interviewers go into an interview hoping to like the candidate, and to find someone to fill an open position. If you have done your homework, you will be ready to answer his or her questions, and to ask some questions of your own, and the interviewer's quest will be over.

Answering Tough Interview Questions

Employers tend to ask potential employees two kinds of questions: directive and open-ended. Directive questions attempt to gain, clarify, or verify factual information. Application forms are a series of directive questions. The open-ended question is an effort to draw out strengths and weaknesses. To deal effectively with all types of interview questions, you need to consider the employer's point of view. No matter what kind of question is asked, an employer really has only three questions:

1. Can you do the work? (Do you have the skills, competence, credentials, and so on?)
2. Will you do the work? (Do you have the motivation and stamina to produce?)
3. Can you get along with others, especially with me, your supervisor? (What are your interpersonal skills and key personality traits?)

When responding to questions, ask yourself: What is the underlying question? This is particularly important with open-ended. It can also help you ferret out potentially discriminatory questions. Accuracy and specificity are the keys to directive questions. The ability to understand yourself as a "product" and to express your strengths will help you answer open-ended questions more effectively.

Here are some questions frequently asked by employers:

▶ Tell me a little about yourself.
▶ Why do you think you are right for this job?
▶ What are your career objectives?
▶ If you could have the perfect position, what would it be?
▶ Do you have plans for continuing education?
▶ Why did you choose this career field?
▶ In what type of position are you most interested?
▶ What do you expect to be doing in five years?
▶ What is your previous work experience? What have you gained or learned from it?
▶ Why are you interested in our organization and in this particular opening?
▶ What salary do you expect to be earning now? In five years?
▶ Why did you choose your particular course of study?
▶ What do you consider to be your major weaknesses? Strengths?
▶ In what ways do you think you can make a contribution to our organization?
▶ What two or three accomplishments have given you the most satisfaction?
▶ Describe your most rewarding college experience.
▶ What have you learned from participation in extracurricular activities?
▶ Are you willing to relocate? Are you willing to travel?
▶ Do you think your grades are a good indication of your academic achievement?
▶ What have you done to show initiative and willingness to work?
▶ What types of books have you read? What journals do you subscribe to?
▶ What jobs have you enjoyed most? Least? Why?

▶ What do you think determines an employee's progress in a good company?

▶ What qualifications make you feel you will be successful in your field?

Asking Questions

Frequently, toward the close of the interview, the interviewer will provide the opportunity to ask questions. Never say that you don't have any questions. This is your chance to set yourself apart from the competition. Prepare your questions in advance. Ask the most important questions first in case there is not enough time to ask all of them. Do not ask questions that might reveal a lack of research. It is inappropriate to ask about salary and benefits unless the employer is offering a position. Most employers do not want to discuss those issues until they are certain you are the right person for the job. Suitable questions include:

▶ What is the typical career path for someone in this position?

▶ What is the realistic time frame for advancement?

▶ How is an employee evaluated and promoted? Is it company policy to promote from within?

▶ What is the retention rate for people in the position for which I am interviewing?

▶ Describe the typical first-year assignments.

▶ Tell me about on-the-job training that is offered.

▶ What are the challenging facets of the job?

▶ What are the opportunities for personal growth?

▶ What are the company's plans for future growth?

▶ What is the company's record of employment stability?

▶ What makes your practice different from your competitors?

▶ What are the company's strengths and weaknesses?

▶ How would you describe your company's personality and management style?

Follow-up Tactics

It is essential to send a letter to thank the interviewer for his or her time. Mention the time and date of the original interview and any important points discussed. Mention any important qualifications that you may have omitted in the interview, and reiterate your interest in the job.

Don't be discouraged if a definite offer is not made at the interview, or if a specific salary is not discussed. The interviewer will usually communicate with her or his office staff or interview other applicants before making an offer. Generally, a decision is reached within a few weeks. If you do not hear from an employer within the time suggested during the interview, follow up with a telephone call. Show your commitment to their timetable. But do show your interest in the position by following up to inquire about a decision.

If you have followed the steps outlined in this book you will soon be choosing between competing job offers. Healthcare is a workers' market at the moment and should continue to be so well into the future. Your main challenge—once you have made the commitment and completed your education—will not be finding job opportunities. It will be making the most of your career and thriving in this demanding but highly rewarding career. The next chapter in this book is dedicated to helping you meet the challenges and find success in your new career.

THE INSIDE TRACK

Who: Susan Parks
What: Nursing Assistant
Where: Norfolk, VA

INSIDER'S STORY

When my mother couldn't live on her own anymore (she had broken her hip and had a partial stroke), my brother and I had to put her in a home. Luckily, we found a wonderful place that was only 15 minutes from my house. I spent many hours at the home with my mother—I was a stay-at-home mom, so I had the opportunity to see her at least five days a week. While I was there, I became very friendly with several of the nursing assistants (NAs) who were my mother's primary caregivers. I really appreciated how much time they spent with my mom each day. They fed her, bathed her, dressed her, took her to physical therapy, kept abreast of her physical and emotional stability, kept her company when I wasn't there, and much more! I watched what they did and thought to myself, "I could do that!"

I've always enjoyed working closely with elderly people—before my children were born, I worked as a receptionist in a geriatric practitioner's office. So, I spoke to a few of the NAs at the home and found out a little more about the job responsibilities, training and certification requirements, and so on. When my youngest child entered kindergarten, I decided to take a training course at a local community college. I got my first job as an NA (with recommendations from my program director and the director of my mom's home, who had seen me care for my mother and interact with the other residents) right after I completed the program and passed my written and oral exams.

I find the job of Nursing Assistant so satisfying because I am helping people who can no longer function on their own. The most difficult part of my job is helping my clients to adjust to life in a residential home—most of them are used to living on their own, being independent. Now, many of them they require help eating, bathing, and getting dressed; they cannot walk on their own; and they need nearly constant supervision so that they don't injure themselves. I also enjoy the companionship aspect of my job—at times, being a stay-at-home mom I missed adult companionship. Now, I not only have my coworkers as friends, I also have a whole new family of residents! I enjoy listening to their wonderful stories about the "good old days," and just spending time with them. The sad part of my job is that some residents' families rarely visit. I try to help them forget by reading to them, getting them involved in new hobbies or activities, and being there to talk to them if they need me.

Sometimes I have to work long or strange hours (like the 6 P.M. to 2 A.M. shift) or complete undesirable tasks (like emptying bedpans) but it is all worthwhile because I am doing something I love and helping people in the meantime. As a Nursing Assistant, you have to be prepared to do some of the grunt work; after all, it is part of your job description. However, the positive aspects of the job—the companionship, the satisfaction in helping someone—definitely outweigh the negative aspects. For most residents, I am their primary caregiver. It's a big responsibility, but also a great joy.

CHAPTER seven

HOW TO SUCCEED ONCE YOU HAVE LANDED THE JOB

IN THIS CHAPTER you will learn how to thrive in your new career position. You will find out about dealing with work relationships, fitting into the workplace culture, managing your time, finding a mentor, and promoting yourself from within the workplace. You will also find information about conquering the challenges particular to a career in healthcare.

YOU HAVE done a lot of hard work to train for and secure a job in your field. Now that you have landed a job, take some time to prepare yourself to excel. If you have followed the steps in this book, you have made a careful choice about your career and you are well trained to meet the demands of your new job. Even so, you might be nervous about your new responsibilities. This chapter will help you cope with the challenges of a new job and give you some pointers about the special challenges you will face working in healthcare.

FITTING INTO THE WORKPLACE CULTURE

Many people are anxious when they start a new job, not only about whether they have the technical skills required, but also about fitting in with coworkers and being accepted by the boss. The good news is that there are practical steps that you can take to fit in and become a member of the team.

Most of these steps are grounded in common sense, but reminding yourself of these basic rules of behavior will help you to feel confident when you arrive for the first day of work at your new job. The most important things you can do to make a good impression are:

▶ Be on time, or even a little early, for work and meetings.
▶ If your job does not require you to wear a uniform, err on the conservative side when you dress for your first day of work.
▶ Do not make personal phone calls at work until you know the policy or general culture of the workplace. Especially in a hospital or doctor's office, phone lines may be required to be free for patients' calls and other medical business.
▶ Strike a balance of formality with your new coworkers—be neither too familiar nor too standoffish.
▶ Take responsibility for your actions, don't take credit for someone else's ideas, and own up to any mistakes you might make. New employees are not expected to be perfect and mistakes are part of the learning curve of a new job. You will make a much better impression if you accept responsibility for your mistakes rather than trying to hide them or pass the blame off onto someone else.
▶ Concentrate on your work rather than on the impression you are making.
▶ If you don't know something, ask someone. Again, you are not expected to know everything about your new workplace. You are better off asking for help than making an unnecessary mistake. Remember that the first few weeks, and sometimes months, on a new job is a learning period.
▶ Don't be offended if coworkers don't warmly include you on the first day. Your coworkers may also be nervous about how you will fit in. Give them time to get to know you.

▶ Help your coworkers if they need it. Don't be afraid to show that you know your stuff!

Two important keys to fitting in at a new job are being open-minded and observant. Every workplace has its own rules and culture. Even if the way things are done seem odd to you at first, do not make a quick judgment. Observe how your coworkers complete their work, how they interact with your supervisor, and how they work together as a team. Use these clues as a guide for your own conduct. Often what seems strange at first will make more sense when you have been on the job longer.

Many institutions give new employees an orientation to make sure they understand the daily routine, such as where to park, as well as policies and procedures of the company. A general orientation can cover just about everything related to the company. Employees are given details about benefits programs, company rules, and perhaps information about the company as a whole. In a department orientation, you will be given more specifics about your job. For some healthcare positions this can be a formal program that can last for a few weeks or up to six months. In smaller medical practices, this orientation might be a more informal introduction to the procedures and responsibilities of your new position provided either by a coworker or a supervisor. The length of any type of orientation depends on the employee's level of training and experience.

Many hospitals or large institutions give helpful classes in areas such as time management, getting along with coworkers, and dealing with ethical issues. Your supervisor can sign you up, or you can sign yourself up, depending on your company's policy. Classes like these are becoming an important supplement to on-the-job training, particularly in the healthcare field.

MANAGING WORK RELATIONSHIPS

Healthcare organizations rely on their employees to get along. A healthcare organization is focused on meeting the needs of patients and employees are expected to work together as a team to provide the best care possible. In some cases, bad relations between employees can lead to serious even fatal errors. While good relations between coworkers are very important, healthcare is a stressful career and this stress can cause difficulties among coworkers. Managing your work relationships increases your own productivity in addition to providing the best care for your patients. Knowledge can be your best tool in getting along with people at work. Learn about other departments—what they do and how their work fits into the work of your department. Learn about the roles played by other people in your department. A good understanding of the structure of your workplace will help you work well with the people who work there. Taking an interest in your coworkers' responsibilities will also indicate that you are a team player.

Here are some tips to help you build positive work relationships:

▶ Always act with integrity; demonstrate that your coworkers can depend on what you say and do.
▶ Work hard and efficiently.
▶ Follow the rules of the workplace—including work hours, dress code, and personal conduct. These rules are created so that employees have an understanding of the company's expectations and so that these expectations are consistent company wide.
▶ Do not ask for any special treatment. Everyone has personal difficulties that sometimes make meeting the demands of a job challenging, but most companies have policies in place to help employees with these situations. Try to resolve any personal problems within the confines of company policy.
▶ Demonstrate your willingness to work as a team.
▶ Have a good attitude and smile often. Particularly if you work directly with patients, a positive attitude can be an important part of caring for patients.
▶ Try to resolve conflicts yourself. If you have a problem with a coworker talk to him or her first, before taking the problem to your supervisor. However, in some situations, including unethical behavior or workplace harassment, it is appropriate to take a problem directly to your boss. In this case, do so discreetly and promptly and do not gossip with your coworkers about the situation.
▶ Keep your work relationships professional. Do not ask personal questions or burden your coworkers with your private troubles. Of course,

you will make friends at work, but during work hours you should try to keep your conversations on a professional level.

▶ Even when you are new to a job and are expected to learn from more experienced coworkers, do not overburden your coworkers. But do try to find a person who is open to helping you, a mentor, and foster that relationship. There is more information later about mentors.

▶ Sincerely thank everyone who does help you, particularly when you are new.

Professionalism is very important for healthcare workers. Because patients trust healthcare workers with their well being, they have high expectations. A patient does not want to be greeted at their doctor's office by a medical assistant who looks messy or disorganized. Nor does a patient recovering from surgery want to be cared for by a nursing assistant who is late for rounds or who has a surly attitude. In order to foster good relations at work, the most important things you can do are maintain the highest standards of professionalism, take your job seriously, and have respect for the work of others.

TIME MANAGEMENT CHALLENGES

Efficiency is key to success in many jobs. As a healthcare worker you will probably find that you are asked to accomplish a lot in a limited amount of time. In some healthcare careers, completing tasks on time can be critical to the health of patients. Time management is an important skill that will contribute to your success in your healthcare career. Some behaviors that contribute to bad time management are:

▶ **Disorganization**. Your inability to complete tasks on time may spring from basic disorganization of workspace and time. If you often stay late, leave unfinished work, or feel there aren't enough hours in the day, disorganization may be to blame. Taking too many breaks, socializing, and inefficient work systems may be at the root of the problem. Lack of motivation can contribute as well.

▶ **Procrastination**. Procrastination may look like disorganization because in both cases you end up finishing tasks late. But the two problems aren't the same. Procrastination springs from one of three main sources: basic dislike of and lack of commitment to the task at hand, fear of not being able to measure up, or misplaced perfectionism.

▶ **Distraction from outside sources**. Distractions lead to a loss of concentration that can spell disaster for your workday. Distractions are very common in some busy healthcare environments, but there are distractions that are of your own making such as personal phone calls, socializing, and non-work-related activity.

▶ **Excessive on-the-job stress**. Stress can contribute to inefficient work habits. Sometimes when people feel overwhelmed, they lose confidence in their abilities and are unable to establish a plan to tackle the work at hand.

TIME MANAGEMENT SOLUTIONS

Fortunately, there are solutions to all the problems outlined above, and more information about coping with stress later in the chapter. Most healthcare jobs from home healthcare workers to surgical technologists require that workers are efficient and organized.

Here are some effective techniques for overcoming the obstacles to good time management.

Conduct a Time Survey

The first step in getting a handle on your time is to understand how you use your time. Over the course of a few days or a week, depending how much your job varies from day to day, keep a detailed log of everything you do on the job. Try to account for every minute of your day. Examine your log and find the places where you wasted valuable time. Do you take a longer lunch break than you thought? Do you spend an hour of your day socializing when you add up all the minutes? The answers to such questions as these can help you make better choices.

Create a To-Do List or Agenda

Schedule yourself to perform your duties in order of importance or time required. Your time survey can also help you make realistic assessments of how much time to leave for certain tasks. One way that people fall behind in their work is that they are unrealistic about the amount of time it will take to accomplish a task. For example, a medical assistant at a doctor's office has to type five reports. If he thinks it only takes 10 minutes to type each report when in fact it takes him 15, he will be 25 minutes behind schedule after five reports. This miscalculation can make planning and therefore time management difficult.

Armed with the information from your time survey, create a list of tasks and the anticipated time it will take to complete each task. Organize the tasks in order of importance, and work through the list over the course of your day. Remember, as you gain experience you will become quicker at tasks. For example, the report that took 15 minutes to type may only take 10 when you have been on the job for several months. Adjust your agendas accordingly.

Use Little Chunks of Time

Always try to make maximum use of your time. If you have five minutes before lunch and you have just finished typing a report, avoid the temptation to wait idly until the five minutes are over. Use the time to take care of a small task on your to-do list such as call a patient or a supplier. You will be amazed at what you can accomplish in five minutes. More important, making the most of your time will give you a sense of control over your day.

Break Large Tasks into Smaller Tasks

Often people procrastinate when a task seems overwhelming. If it seems like you will never complete an impossibly large project, why even start? To prevent inertia, break a large project into smaller manageable tasks. For example, if you have been asked to enter all the patients' records into a computer database, tackle the job one letter of the alphabet at a time. Only put the A's on your list. When you finish with the A's, put the B's on your list and so on.

Reward Yourself

If you are working on a big task or on a difficult project, treat yourself after you have completed a portion of the project. Reward yourself for your accomplishments; it will help you to stay motivated and keep your attitude positive.

Eat Properly, Exercise, and Get Enough Sleep

You may be surprised to learn that boredom and lack of productivity at work often stem from poor health habits, both on and off the job. Getting enough sleep at night is probably the single most important step you can take to improve your work performance. If you are tired, everything seems harder because your energy is low. Skipping breakfast and eating junk food for lunch and dinner has a similar effect. Healthy food eaten in moderate amounts will greatly increase your energy level and productivity. Exercise also increases your energy. Keeping to a regular program of exercise will help you feel more lively and focused.

Alternate Tasks to Add Variety

If you have some say in how you spend your time at work, add variety to your day by changing from one task to another rather than working on one job past the point of boredom. You shouldn't flip-flop compulsively, of course; but changing to another task when you have reached your capacity with another will help you get both tasks completed faster.

Take Mini-Breaks

Sitting in one place, in one position, for long periods can be stultifying. But some healthcare jobs do not allow workers to move about or alternate tasks. Taking unobtrusive mini-breaks will not only alleviate body strain but aid relaxation, which helps reduce stress and improve productivity. Here are some simple mini-breaks:

- ▶ Stand up and stretch a moment, then sit back down.
- ▶ Yawn and blink (these also help release tension and lubricate eyes).
- ▶ Massage your hands and fingers or cover your eyes with your palms.
- ▶ Take several deep, controlled breaths.
- ▶ Do isometric exercises, such as calf flexes, ankle twirls, stomach tightening and relaxation, gentle shoulder shrugs, and head-rolls.
- ▶ Stretch while remaining seated; clasp your hands behind your head and pull your shoulders way back (this is called the executive stretch).

Rearrange Your Workstation

If you find yourself distracted by others—either because people tend to stop at your desk to chat or because they bump into your desk as they pass—it's best to reposition your workstation, if you are allowed to do so. You may want to turn so that you face a wall or window, so that you aren't facing into oncoming traffic. Also arrange your workstation for maximum efficiency. Make sure that the things you need most often are the easiest to reach and those items that you only use occasionally are out of the way.

DEALING WITH YOUR BOSS

Establishing a good working relationship with your supervisor may be the most important thing you can do to succeed at your new job. After all, it is your supervisor who evaluates your performance and it is his or her opinion that really counts when you are interested in getting a raise or being promoted. Working well with your boss will also make your day-to-day work life rewarding and agreeable.

Many of the work habits about which you have already read apply to getting along with your boss. Being an efficient and capable worker are the most important ingredients in making a successful relationship. But there are other things that you can do to help foster this important relationship, including:

▶ Defer to your boss's judgment. If you boss asks you to do something, or asks you to change the priority of your tasks, do as you have been asked. Do not question your boss's judgment, especially when you are establishing a relationship. Sometimes when you have worked for someone for a period of time, that person will come to rely on your judgment and value your input, but you have to build up this respect.

▶ Learn to accept criticism. If your immediate supervisor is a doctor or an administrator in a busy medical practice, you may need to develop a bit of a thick skin. Hospitals and doctors' offices are often stressful environments and your supervisor may be under a great deal of pressure. In this case, sometimes supervisors do not have the time to explain carefully and kindly a problem or mistake. If you can learn not to take sharp or abrupt criticism personally and simply correct the mistake, your boss will appreciate your maturity and ability to handle yourself under stress.

▶ Make your boss a priority. For example, if you are on the phone and your boss comes over to your desk, try to finish the conversation as quickly as possible so that you can turn your attention to your boss.

▶ Establish good communication with your boss. Especially if you work for a busy doctor, determine a good time of day to check in and go over any work issues or to give a progress report. Try not to go to your boss with every little question. Store up your questions and present them in an organized manner at a time when your boss has time to give you his or her attention. It is important to keep your boss up to date on your work and to make sure that you are in agreement about priorities.

Even though you do work well with your boss, you should not be expected to take the brunt of his or her stress. It is your job to help your boss take care of patients and run a successful medical practice, but this does not mean that you have to sacrifice yourself for that goal. Here are keys to resisting pressure from your supervisors:

- ▶ Remember that you have a life outside work, and don't let work overrun your outside life. Talk to your boss if you need to make some adjustments, but make sure when you raise a problem that you have a positive solution in mind.
- ▶ Set limits, even with your boss. Again good communication is the key to setting reasonable limits.
- ▶ Learn physical relaxation techniques. You will learn more about coping with stress later in this chapter.

INTERNAL PRESSURE

Often, the greatest pressure we have to bear is that which we put on ourselves. This can sometimes be a positive motivating force, but it can reach bullying proportions if we let it. Here are three ways to relieve unreasonable pressure from within:

- ▶ Weed out perfectionism—care more about overall excellence than minor details.
- ▶ Care more about the quality of your work than about what others (including your boss) think of you.
- ▶ Be nice to yourself. Remember to dwell on the positive in your work not the negative. Don't beat yourself up for mistakes. Accept them, correct them, and move on.

FINDING A MENTOR

One of your best resources at work is a good mentor. A mentor can help you greatly while you learn about your new job, get acquainted with your new building, and begin to adjust to your work surroundings. He or she also may teach you things about your job that you didn't learn in school.

Some hospitals and medical practices have established mentoring programs, in which a new staff member is assigned to a more experienced worker—sometimes called a resource person. If this is not the case at your job, you can find an informal mentor. Who is a good mentor?

▶ a person who takes an interest in your career
▶ a person who has knowledge to pass along to you
▶ a person who is a good listener
▶ a person who you feel comfortable going to for advice

A mentor can be a coworker, your supervisor, someone in another department, an alumnus/a from your training program who works at the same medical facility, in short, anyone who fits the description above. A mentor is a good sounding board when you are not sure how to approach a problem at work. If your mentor is further along the career ladder, he or she can offer career advice and inform you about industry trends. A mentor can also let you know about opportunities and help you expand your network.

PROMOTING YOURSELF

Many times in your career you will have chances to promote yourself to a higher-level position or an improved work situation. Before you ask for a promotion, show your employer or supervisor that you have dedicated yourself to your current position, you have performed well, your attendance is satisfactory, you have been cooperative and flexible, and you have gained the necessary training.

Hospitals usually hire entry-level workers for a contract position. You may be hired as a nurse's aide and be required to keep that position for six months before requesting a promotion or schedule change. You should only accept the job if you can commit to these terms. A nursing recruiter from Athens, Georgia, explains:

> We tell applicants, "These are the hours of this position. Is there any-
> thing that would prevent you from working these hours?" We've got to
> know if the person's going to be able to work the hours. Some people
> will say they want days but they will take nights. Well, we try not to
> do that because when you are hired into a night position, you are
> committed to that, and a lot of times, those people start applying
> right away to change to days. You can't do that. Don't take the
> job just to get your foot in the door.

After six months you are eligible to transfer if you have the qualifications and if your employment record is clean. You will need to fill out a job transfer request form explaining to your supervisor and others when and why you wish to transfer. You won't get promoted if you have performance or attendance problems.

Private practices and group practices hire different numbers of staff and have different work policies. You may be promoted as soon as you receive the training needed for a promotion, if the physician feels you can do the work. In these cases, it is up to the employer. Hospitals follow more formal guidelines for promotions.

As you learned in Chapter 1, additional training is often the key to career advancement. However, in addition to having the right level of training, you need to have performed well in your current position. Consistently maintaining high professional standards, meeting and exceeding the requirements of your position, fostering good communications, and having a positive attitude will all contribute to gaining a promotion.

MEETING THE CHALLENGES OF HEALTHCARE CAREERS

Working in healthcare is a particularly rewarding career because you are providing a valuable service and helping to improve the quality of other people's lives. Most healthcare workers get a great deal of satisfaction out of knowing that they are helping others. However, healthcare is also a career that comes with special challenges. One reason for the abundant opportunity in certain healthcare fields is worker burnout. Mental exhaustion is a common factor that causes people to leave the profession.

The good news is that there are numerous strategies for coping with stress and burnout and other trials faced by healthcare workers. If you are prepared to meet these challenges you can enjoy the tremendous rewards of these careers.

Coping with Stress

As in many other careers, healthcare workers face the stress of having too much to do, not having enough time, dealing with stressed-out bosses, and coping with difficult coworkers. In addition, healthcare workers often work with patients who are in pain, depressed, or angry and who take these feelings out on their caregivers. There is also the stress of working in life-and-death situations. For many office workers a mistake can be corrected without serious consequences or at worse some money is lost. But some healthcare workers have the added pressure of making a potentially deadly mistake. For example, a transcription error in a report could result in inaccurate medical records that could result in a fatal misdiagnosis.

These challenges are also what make healthcare work so rewarding. Bringing a smile to a depressed patient's face or knowing that lives depend on your work can be great motivators. However, there are several methods that help you deal with stress so that it does not interfere with your work, including:

- ▶ Keep a positive attitude. Envision positive outcomes of your work. For example, instead of dreading an encounter with an angry patient, try to imagine that your cheerful attitude will lessen the patient's anger.
- ▶ Learn to eliminate guilt. Guilt is a negative emotion that takes away your motivation.
- ▶ Set boundaries. Determine the workload that you can reasonably handle and do not accept more work than you can successfully accomplish. You may need to work with your supervisor to set an appropriate workload.
- ▶ Let your frustration out. Talk out your stresses with a trusted friend, preferably not a coworker. Venting with coworkers can sometimes add

to stress because it contributes to a negative work environment. It may also help to write down the causes of your stress. It might help you put things in perspective and find solutions.

▶ Enjoy yourself at work. Laugh whenever you get the chance—laughter is a great stress reliever. If, for example, you are a home health aide, listen to music that energizes you in your car as you drive from one job to the next.

▶ Develop friendly relationships at work so you have a strong support network among your coworkers.

Working the Night Shift

Many healthcare providers work a schedule other than the traditional 9-to-5 workday. Particularly when you are starting out, you may be required to work at night. Day shifts are sometimes reserved for more experienced personnel. This can be physically and emotionally demanding. Sleep deprivation is one of the greatest dangers of working the night shift, and lack of sleep is a leading cause of stress. Fortunately, there are ways to cope with leading a nocturnal life.

▶ Get uninterrupted sleep during the day. Make sure your family and friends respect that you are not "napping" because you are sleeping during the day. Create a dark, quiet environment that allows you to get a good "day's" sleep.

▶ If, for example, your family responsibilities make it difficult for you to get uninterrupted sleep during the day, take naps during your breaks at work. Studies show that 15- to 25-minute naps can significantly revive you. Hospitals often have places where workers can take a quick nap because of the long and irregular working hours that are expected.

▶ Watch your caffeine and sugar. Caffeine is an effective reviver but if you overindulge it can affect your sleep. The stimulating effects of caffeine can last up to seven hours, so workers who drink coffee to get them through the end of a long night will sacrifice the much-needed sleep at the end of their shift. Sugar is only a temporary reviver and has an overall tiring effect. Sugar gives you a quick boost of energy, but when your body burns up the sugar's energy it is more depleted of energy than before you ate the sugar. A complex carbohydrate snack is a much better choice to give you the energy to get through the end of your shift.

▶ Avoid alcohol as a sleep aid. Some people will have a drink or two to help them unwind before going to bed. The alcohol does help you fall asleep, but results in less restful sleep.

▶ Try to develop a regular sleep pattern. Even on your days off, do not try to switch to a day schedule. Of course, you will want to spend time with your family and friends who are on a day schedule. Do not completely abandon your schedule, but instead adjust your hours. Much like "day people" who stay up late and sleep in on weekends, you can shift your hours on your days off without completely giving up your established sleep pattern. Regular hours are one of the key factors in getting healthy restful sleep.

▶ Try to see a little daylight each day. Sunlight can be an important factor in mental well being, so before or after your shift, try to spend some time outdoors.

▶ Stay involved with your family and friends even if you are on different schedules. Keeping communication open can help prevent night shift workers from feeling isolated. E-mail is a good way to keep in touch because it is not dependent on time. You may not be able to call your friend at 3:00 A.M. but you can send an e-mail message whenever you have the time. If you have a family, create a system like a bulletin board for notes and pictures that will keep you in the loop when your face-to-face time is limited.

▶ Be creative with your time. If you miss nights out with your spouse, make a date to go out for breakfast at a special restaurant. Find ways to enjoy your unusual hours. Being on the opposite schedule from many people means that you do not have to fight traffic, or crowded supermarkets, for example. You can take advantage of early bird specials and you can learn about the night sky. You might even develop an appreciation for the "night life."

Fighting Burnout

Along with stress itself, burnout—the end result of unmanaged stress—is a leading cause of people leaving the healthcare profession. Burnout is the set of physical and emotional symptoms that result from the cumulative effects of stress. Essentially you can prevent burnout if you learn to manage your stress following some of the strategies already discussed.

However, because burnout can lead to poor job performance and a severe lack of motivation, it is important to learn how to recognize the warning signs of burnout and how to prevent your case from getting any worse. The point at which a person will become burnt out varies from person to person—much like there are people who lose their tempers easily and some people who never lose their cool. Everyone has his or her own threshold, and it is important to know yours. Some warning signs of burnout include:

▶ difficulty summoning energy or enthusiasm for work
▶ need for longer recovery time—for example, a weekend is no longer sufficient to feel rested and ready to face the challenges of the workplace
▶ negative mood at the beginning of the day—dread at facing the day
▶ negative mood at the end of the day—only recollections of work are negative incidents
▶ physical symptoms such as increased blood pressure and insomnia
▶ mental symptoms such as depression or dependence on drugs or alcohol

There are degrees of burnout—ranging from general negativity about work to a strong desire to quit working. It is important to catch burnout at the early stages before you get to the point when you can't stand the thought of working another day. Here are some steps you can take to fight burnout at the first warning signs:

▶ Depend on your colleagues for support. Seek your colleagues' advice when you are in a difficult situation. Your coworkers can be a source of positive feedback who will help reinforce your sense of purpose.
▶ Talk through your problems with a friend, trusted colleague, or supervisor. Sometimes simply sounding out your problems can help clarify the situation.

▶ Seek professional counseling if you feel your case of burnout has become severe. A professional counselor can work with you to examine what motivates you and help you to set goals and priorities.

▶ Evaluate your priorities and make sure you are meeting your needs. First rank the areas of your life in terms of the percent of your energy you invest in each area such as family, career, friends, hobbies, volunteer work, education, physical fitness, and so on. Then rank each area again with the percent you would like to devote to each area. Make adjustments in your schedule that allow you to meet, or at least approach, your ideal percentages.

Some people are more vulnerable to burnout than others. Personalities at a high risk for burnout include people who:

▶ have trouble saying "no"
▶ take on more work than they can handle
▶ don't set boundaries and allow work to overtake their personal lives
▶ suppress their emotions
▶ have a negative self-image
▶ have difficulty managing stress or allow stress to accumulate

If you recognize yourself in the profile there are steps you can take to make yourself less vulnerable. Recognizing that you have these tendencies is half the battle. If you realize that you always say "yes" when you are asked to do more than you can handle, you can watch for this situation and start to say "no." The most important key to preventing burnout is to recognize it early and to take the necessary steps to nip it in the bud.

FINAL THOUGHTS

Every career comes with risks; for healthcare workers among the greatest risks are stress and burnout. However, you can prevent these factors from harming your career by taking steps to manage stress before it gets out of control. With the risks come rewards, and healthcare is one of the most rewarding careers. There are very few other professions that have such an immediate and crucial impact on the quality of other people's lives. A healthcare worker makes a tremendous difference in the lives of the patients he or she treats—whether directly or indirectly.

Your career is in your hands. You can manage your career so that it meets your needs and provides continuing challenges and rewards. The steps outlined in this book are aimed at helping you get started in your new career, but much of the advice is equally applicable to taking the next step—perhaps getting additional training so you can achieve the next level in your chosen field. One thing is certain, the opportunities in the healthcare field will continue to grow and provide new challenges for workers.

THE INSIDE TRACK

Who: Kelly Lee
What: Sonography Technician
Where: Brookline, Massachusetts

INSIDER'S STORY

I have been working as a sonography technician at an OB/GYN private practice for almost four years. I work with a group of eight doctors, as well as several nurse practitioners and nurses, which makes for a very busy office.

Mostly, I work with the sonogram equipment and perform the sonogram on patients. I always take the time to explain the procedure to the patient before we actually get started because many women are nervous about what to expect. I also ensure that the patient has followed pre-visit procedures and has provided me with her full medical history before beginning the sonogram.

Once I have the patient informed and reasonably comfortable, I begin to scan images to capture for the doctor. I try to get clear shots at all the right angles while working quickly so that the process is not too time-consuming. I also check out the equipment after the procedure is finished so that I know that I'll be set up properly for the next patient.

For training, I attended a two-year program in Massachusetts, and I graduated with an associate's degree in Diagnostic Medical Sonography. Aside from my classroom education, I would say that the most important skill to have in this field is an eye for detail. Performing sonograms and searching for tiny irregularities requires my full attention and concentration. I know that my job is vital to patients' and their babies' health, and I take my role very seriously. If I miss something in my scan, and if it doesn't get captured on my screen shots, the doctor will not know about a possible issue and steps may not get taken in a timely manner. Any day that a potential problem goes unnoticed can mean the difference between life and death.

One of the hardest parts of the job is to remain neutral. Many women who I see are pregnant and anxious about information that I see as I perform the sonogram. Others are anxious about the status of a possible tumor or irregularity, and they often ask me what I'm finding in the images. I am not at liberty to tell the patient any specifics—that's the doctor's role. Though I am confident in my skills at recognizing what I see in the sonogram, the news is not mine to deliver, good or bad. I strive to be careful not to let potentially bad news show on my face. Being discreet, courteous, and professional is my priority.

I recommend a solid two-year program as a minimum. Some schools give a one-year certificate, but I think that a college program provides better experience. Also, taking classes in other areas helped me to develop my communication skills, especially in writing, and my people skills, too. The other piece of advice I have is to understand that working in a busy office requires diplomacy and flexibility. I enjoy working in this practice, but it can get very hectic, and tempers can flare up and frustration can show. It's best to remember that I'm here to do a job and I need to concentrate on it first, not on office gossip or trying to avoid the office manager if she's having a bad day. On the other hand, there is great camaraderie that develops in a fast-paced office. I have learned a lot about my job function, as well as about career development.

CHAPTER eight

CAREERS IN GERONTOLOGY

ALTHOUGH EVERY area of healthcare career market shows very favorable signs of growth in the upcoming years, gerontology shows the greatest promise. In this chapter you will learn all about careers in eldercare, from areas of specialization to employers to specific training programs. You will also learn about the challenges and rewards of this avenue in the healthcare careers.

THE U.S. POPULATION is growing older. A rising demographic tide of aging baby boomers—those born between 1946 and 1964—and increased longevity have made adults age 65 and older the fastest growing segment of today's population. Projected within the next 30 years, this "elder boom" will dramatically influence the field of healthcare, creating new jobs throughout the industry. Consider these population trends:

- ▶ In 2030, the population of adults age 65 and older will be nearly twice as large as it is today. By then, an estimated 70 million people will be over age 65.
- ▶ People are living longer than ever due to healthier lifestyles and improved medical care. In the United States, average life expectancy (the

number of years one can expect to live) has increased more in the past 100 years than in the previous 2,000.

▶ The older population is getting older. Today, the percentage of Americans age 85 and older is 34 times larger than it was in 1900. And experts predict this trend to continue, making the "oldest old" the fastest-growing age group.

As older adults make up an increasing proportion of the healthcare caseload, the demand for eldercare providers is growing as well. Job opportunities throughout the healthcare industry are expanding for people with a variety of skills and educational levels. Senior citizens who wish to continue to be active and live independently will require healthcare services outside of the traditional hospital or nursing home setting. Health promotion activities, disease prevention efforts, and home healthcare will increase. Home healthcare services, which provide medical, nursing, and personal care to elders in their own homes, is one of the fastest growing industries in the U.S. economy. Employment in home healthcare is projected to increase 80 percent through 2008, compared to an average of 15 percent for all industries.

Although older adults are healthier than ever, physical challenges often increase with age. Impaired hearing and changes in vision can result from the normal aging process. In addition, a number of medical conditions occur more frequently in older adults, such as arthritis, hypertension (high blood pressure), heart disease, cataracts, diabetes, prostate problems, osteoporosis, and stroke. Chronic conditions and disease can limit a person's ability to function. Currently, an estimated 30 percent of older adults report that their activities are limited by chronic conditions, and more than half report having at least one disability. Many elderly adults require some kind of assistance ranging from help around the house to 24-hour access to skilled nursing care.

While older adults make up a diverse group, they often share health, social, emotional, and economic needs. Gerontology is an emerging field that studies and seeks to address those needs. Currently, you do not need a background in gerontology to begin a career providing care to older adults. However, as the elderly population demands more and more healthcare and other services, job seekers with a knowledge and understanding of the issues that affect this age group will have a competitive advantage.

What Is Gerontology?

Gerontology is a growing field that studies and addresses the physical, mental, emotional, and social changes that are often a part of the aging process. Gerontology is a multidisciplinary field that includes professionals in medicine, nursing, social work, law, public policy, architecture, adult education, among others. For example, an architect who specializes in the design and construction of assisted living facilities may consider herself a gerontologist. Similarly, a dietitian who plans meals at a nursing home may also be a gerontologist. The term "geriatrics" refers more specifically to the study of disease in later life and the healthcare of older adults.

HOT JOBS

Demand is increasing for eldercare workers in a wide range of health services. According to the National Institute on Aging, the aging of the population will spur a growing need for a variety of specialists including audiologists (those who treat people with hearing problems), geriatric care nurses, psychologists, and physical, occupational, and speech therapists.

However, you don't have to be a specialist to provide needed health services to the elderly. If you're interested in working with older patients, there are a number of entry-level healthcare jobs from which to choose. The U.S. Bureau of Labor projects high-growth levels for the occupations listed below. Some of these jobs do not require specialized training beyond high school. For more details about job duties and training requirements, refer to Chapter 1.

Home Health Aides

Home health aide is among the top ten fastest-growing occupations in the healthcare industry due to the increase of home care for the aging population. Providing care for elderly patients in their homes is a rising trend for several reasons. It is less expensive than hospital care or long-term care in a nursing home and in many instances, is more effective because the patient feels more comfortable in his or her own environment. Improvements in medical technology have also contributed to the development of in-home treatments. Personal care and home health aides assist the elderly with activities of daily living such as bathing, dressing, and eating. They may provide some housekeeping, shop for groceries, and plan and prepare meals. In addition, they may help administer medications and assist with prescribed exercises.

Nursing Assistants

The employment of nursing assistants will increase faster than average for all occupations due to the long-term care needs of the growing elderly population. Long-term care units include nursing homes and residential care facilities. Currently, one-half of all nursing assistants work in nursing homes, providing much of the daily, hands-on care to elderly residents. Nursing assistants (also called geriatric assistants) employed by nursing homes must be certified, which means that they must complete 75 hours of training and pass a competency evaluation program.

Physical Therapy Assistants and Aides

The demand for physical therapy assistants and aides will rise as the baby-boom generation ages and the incidence for heart attack, stroke, fractures, arthritis, and other injuries and illnesses increase. Physical therapy, which aims to improve mobility and relieve pain, will help improve the quality of life for many older Americans with disabling conditions. Physical therapy assistants help with prescribed exercises and perform treatments such as massages, electrical stimulation, paraffin baths, and other therapies under the direction of a physical therapist. Most licensed physical therapy assistants have an associate's degree. Physical therapy aides perform a more limited range of tasks, such as keeping the treatment area clean, assisting a patient in moving to and from the treatment area, and clerical work. Aides receive training on the job.

Occupational Therapy Assistants and Aides

Occupational therapy assistants and aides will be instrumental in helping senior citizens maintain active, independent lifestyles. Employment for occupational therapy assistants and aides is projected to grow faster than average for all occupations as the older population increases and needs their services. The goal of occupational therapy is to help individuals with mental, emotional, or physical impairment function in their daily environment.

Occupational therapy assistants and aides work under the supervision of occupational therapists to help patients perform a range of routine tasks from using a computer to dressing, cooking, or eating. Assistants may teach a person the proper method to move from a bed to a wheelchair or provide exercises that improve an elderly person's strength and flexibility. Occupational therapy assistants must complete an associate's degree or certificate program. Occupational therapy aides perform a range of clerical tasks such as scheduling appointments or completing paperwork. They also prepare equipment used during treatment. Aides are trained on the job.

Respiratory Therapists

Older adults suffer more from respiratory ailments and diseases such as pneumonia, chronic bronchitis, emphysema, and heart disease—all of which can require respiratory services—than the general population. Job opportunities for respiratory therapists will increase much faster than the average for all occupations because of the substantial growth of the middle-aged and elderly population. Hospitals continue to employ about 90 percent of all respiratory therapists, but a growing number will work with elderly patients in home health agencies and nursing homes. In home care, therapists inspect and clean life-support systems and teach patients and their families know how to use equipment properly.

OTHER CAREER OPTIONS

If you're not sure you want to be a direct caregiver, you might consider working in a setting that provides services for the aging. Nursing homes, offices of physicians who specialize in geriatric medicine, adult day centers, and other groups and organizations hire *medical assistants*, *receptionists*, and other *administrative support* staff.

The following job descriptions will give you an idea about other job opportunities in elder health services. Entry-level assistant positions generally require an associate's degree at a minimum. Advancement usually requires job experience and additional education.

- ▶ **Administrators and managers** oversee the day-to-day operation of facilities that care for the aging, such as nursing homes or adult day centers.
- ▶ **Geriatric care managers** are professionals who assess an older person's living environment and aid families with long-term care planning. They may work directly for a family or individual or for a hospital or health maintenance organization.
- ▶ **Marketing specialists** develop marketing and advertising strategies in order to sell health services to the older population. They may work for a nursing home, hospital, retirement community, social service agency, or health maintenance organization.
- ▶ **Program coordinators and activities directors** plan health promotion and recreation activities at nursing homes, assisted living facilities, and senior centers.

TYPES OF EMPLOYERS

Whether you work with elderly patients or with patients of all ages may depend on your employer. For example, a nursing assistant at a community hospital works with patients of all ages, whereas a nursing assistant at an assisted living facility focuses entirely on elderly care. The following are some types of employers that specialize in health services for older adults.

Nursing homes provide three basic levels of long-term care for elderly patients. A *residential care facility* provides independent, apartment-style living with a minimum of medical monitoring. This type of facility often offers a central dining area and housekeeping services. An *intermediate care facility* offers meals and increased nursing care for seniors who can no longer live independently. A *skilled nursing facility* provides 24-hour access to nursing care, physician coverage, and rehabilitation services to elders who need continuous care. All three types offer fitness and social activities. The term *assisted living facility* usually refers to a residential care facility that offers a range of nursing care based on each resident's level of need. Some assisted living facilities include all three of the types of care described above, so that if an active senior becomes ill or disabled, he or she can move into a skilled nursing wing in the same establishment.

Home health and personal care agencies place aides in patients' homes to provide nursing and personal care services. Although patients may be of any age, many are elderly adults. Care may include housekeeping or assisting patients with activities of daily living such as bathing, dressing, or walking. Aides may also give medications or assist with medical equipment such as ventilators that help patients breathe. Aides work under the supervision of a nurse or physical therapist.

Geriatric medicine practices are group practices of physicians who specialize in healthcare for older adults.

Senior centers serve active older adults and those who may have minor problems with mobility and activities of daily living. These community-based centers provide a variety of health-related programs and social activities.

Adult day services (also called *adult daycare*) are community-based programs that serve older adults with serious mobility limitations or medical conditions that require daily attention. Adult day programs generally operate during normal business hours five days a week, although some are open in the evenings or weekends. These programs often provide a range of services including nursing care, rehabilitation therapy, personal care, meals, transportation, and social activities.

Although *hospitals* provide medical care to people of all ages, many patients are elderly—they account for 36% of all hospital stays. Also, a growing number of hospitals run long-term care facilities or offer home healthcare services to meet the needs of the aging population.

Hospices provide medical, emotional, and spiritual care to terminally ill patients and their families. Some hospices are freestanding institutions; some are special units in a hospital. Often, a healthcare team provides hospice services in a patient's home. Although terminally ill patients include people of all ages, most receiving hospice care are elderly—more than 70 percent are age 65 and older.

Other potential employers include *public health and welfare departments, recreation departments, aging associations,* and *retirement communities.*

Location, Location

Today, the state of Pennsylvania tops the chart for nursing-home job opportunities. Nursing home establishments in that state hire over 31,000 workers. The other top five states for employees of continuing care facilities are Ohio, California, Florida, and Illinois. If you don't already live in one of these states, do you need to relocate in order to land a job serving the elderly? Not at all. As baby boomers reach retirement age in 2011, the size of the elderly population will increase in all states. By 2025, the elderly will constitute over 15 percent of the population in 48 states. California will still rank first in having the largest age-65-and-over population, followed by Florida. Alaska will have the smallest elderly group, making up 10 percent of the population.

TRAINING AND EDUCATION

Currently over 1,500 schools offer courses in gerontology. Programs in the field of the aging range from continuing education classes to degree programs at the associate level and higher. Whether or not you complete an instructional program—and what kind of program you choose—depends on your personal interests and job objectives. Generally, professionals in gerontology are not licensed or certified in the field, although this may change as the field expands to meet the needs of a growing elderly population. Even jobs that provide direct care to the aging do not require special training or education in gerontology. For example, a physical therapy assistant who works with nursing home residents is not required to have a background in gerontology. Because nursing assistants and home health aides often care for elderly patients, training programs for these occupations usually incorporate a basic introduction to geriatric care, but additional training in gerontology is not essential.

Although a background in gerontology is not currently required to work with the aging, keep in mind that knowledge about the aging process and awareness of issues that affect older patients can give you a competitive edge in the job market. An understanding of the physical, emotional, mental, and social needs of elderly patients can impress potential employers and provide you with valuable job skills. And, as the elderly make up an increasing proportion of patients, the demand for nurses, nursing assistants, and other health service providers with expertise in gerontology will likely grow.

Continuing Education

Classes in gerontology are often non-credit courses, often called continuing education classes, that can assist students who are preparing for a new career or people who are already working and wish to gain knowledge about the age group that they serve. Some continuing education classes can be applied toward a degree program. Many institutions including technical schools, colleges, universities, aging associations, hospitals, nursing homes, and job training firms offer courses in gerontology. Continuing education in gerontology may also fulfill course requirements to maintain a license or certificate in nursing. For example, all certified nursing homes in the United States require that nursing assistants receive at least 12 hours of education annually.

Degree Programs

Training programs in gerontology that lead to a degree vary in focus. Some schools offer students the option of choosing gerontology as a specialty area within a larger course of study. For example, a student of psychology who plans to work with older patients may earn a degree in psychology with a specialization, or minor, in gerontology. Degree programs in sociology, medicine, nursing, social work, and healthcare administration sometimes offer a specialization in gerontology.

Other schools offer a degree or major in gerontology. Community college programs are increasingly offering associate-level degrees in gerontology. These programs may be attractive to students who are seeking entry-level positions in healthcare administration in nursing homes, assisted living centers, aging associations, or other institutions that care for the elderly. A degree program may also appeal to nurses, nursing assistants, and other health service providers who currently work with the elderly and wish to increase their job marketability and skills.

Sample Program Description

Here is a program description of a two-year A.A.S. (associate in applied science) degree in gerontology offered by the University of Arkansas at Fort Smith. This program prepares students for entry-level positions in public and private agencies that provide health, social, or psychological services to the aging. The first two semesters of the program include general education courses in English, college algebra, computer applications, general psychology, and nutrition. The remaining two semesters focus on the study of gerontology. Here is a partial course description:

GERO 1203 Introduction to Gerontology—A study of the aging process in the United States. Presents the physical and mental realities of growing older, the economics of aging, living arrangements of older people, social support systems, older people at risk, and public policy.

GERO 1243 Biology and Physiology of Aging—A study of the human body and body functions during the aging process.

GERO 2423 Ethnic and Cultural Diversity in the Aging Populations— Presents multicultural perspectives and ethical implications in aging.

GERO 2463 Drug Use and Abuse—Teaches students to recognize the kinds of drugs that are used and abused by the elderly, what they do to the body, and the behaviors associated with their abuse.

Source: The University of Arkansas at Forth Smith, www.uafortsmith.edu.

The program includes hands-on experience working with both well-functioning older adults and those with health challenges. It also offers on-site experience at nursing homes or other service agencies in areas of professional management and program development.

Tuition at the University of Arkansas at Fort Smith is currently $41 per hour for county residents, $52 for in-state residents, and $102 for out-of-state residents. For more information about healthcare training programs, see Chapter 3.

CHALLENGES AND REWARDS

In addition to expanding career options, the field of gerontology offers many opportunities for personal and professional growth. Eldercaregivers enjoy the satisfaction of helping older adults stay healthy; meet physical, mental, and emotional challenges; and improve the overall quality of their lives. Providing care to the aging population also gives workers insight about elderly friends and relatives in their personal lives as well as an understanding about their own aging process. Here are some of the other challenges and rewards a job in gerontology can offer:

▶ **Relationships**—Direct caregivers often develop satisfying, caring relationships with the patients they serve. Because nursing homes offer long-term care, employees in these establishments may enjoy ongoing relationships with patients over months or years. Working with the elderly can also be emotionally demanding. Some patients can be pleasant and cooperative while others are more difficult. Learning to deal with death and loss may be a part of the job. Many of those who work with elderly adults enjoy the wealth of experience, wit, and creativity their patients offer.

▶ **Working environment**—Work settings can differ widely. In delivering home care, employees may need to adapt to a variety of environments. Some may be clean and pleasant, others may be less accommodating. Being able to work in different settings while maintaining a discreet, respectful attitude in someone's home are a requisite for providing home healthcare.

▶ **Teamwork**—Providing care and services to the elderly requires both coordination and collaboration. If you are a direct caregiver, you will most likely work as part of a healthcare team that may include nurses, physicians, physical or occupational therapists, social workers, and counselors. If you are a service provider, you may coordinate with housing agencies, transportation providers, nurses, and family counselors. Because gerontology involves many professionals outside of the healthcare field, you may be exposed to a number of other disciplines such as law, adult education, or architecture.

▶ **Advancement**—Advancement opportunities vary by job, employer, and skill and educational level. Entry-level workers providing direct care may advance to higher-level positions or to new occupations with experience and in some cases, further education and training. Larger establishments, such as hospitals or nursing facilities, usually offer a greater range of opportunities. Because gerontology is an emerging field, it offers room for innovation and development of new ideas, services, and products.

IS A CAREER IN ELDERCARE RIGHT FOR YOU?

If you're interested in pursuing a career in eldercare, how do you know if you're suited to the work? Most caregivers are motivated by a desire to help people and do not mind tasks that can be routine and sometimes unpleasant. Personality traits of successful caregivers include respect for older adults, a sense of responsibility, compassion, and a cheerful, positive attitude. Caregivers should be in good health. Some states require that health service providers complete a physical examination and a tuberculosis test.

Because eldercare is an area of specialization within many of the career choices discussed earlier in the book, you might elect to serve this population of patients at any point in your career. One thing is certain. Healthcare workers who make gerontology the focus of their careers will not only be rewarded with excellent job prospects but also with the satisfaction that they are performing a vital function in society.

RELATED ASSOCIATIONS

The following are some associations that you can contact for further information about aging issues as well as job opportunities in gerontology.

American Association of Retired Persons (AARP)
601 E Street NW
Washington, DC 20049
800-424-3410

American Society on Aging (ASA)
833 Market Street, Suite 511
San Francisco, CA 94103-1824
415-974-9600

Association for Gerontology in Higher Education (AGHE)
1030 15th Street NW, Suite 240
Washington, DC 20005-1503
202-289-9806

Gerontological Society of America (GSA)
1030 15th Street NW, Suite 250
Washington, DC 20005
202-842-1275

National Association of Area Agencies on Aging (NAAAA)
927 15th Street NW, 6th Floor
Washington, DC 20005
202-296-8130

National Association of State Units on Aging (NASUA)
1225 Eye Street NW, Suite 725
Washington, DC 20005
202-898-2578

National Council on the Aging (NCOA)
409 Third Street SW, Suite 200
Washington, DC 20024
202-479-1200

National Institute on Aging (NIA)
Building 31, Room 5C27
31 Center Drive, MSC 2292
Bethesda, MD 20892
301-496-1752

U.S. Administration on Aging (AoA)
330 Independence Avenue SW
Washington, DC 20201
202-619-7501

U.S. Census Bureau
Age and Sex Statistics Branch
Population Division
Washington, DC 20233
301-457-2378

THE INSIDE TRACK

Who: Clyde Goodall

What: Occupational Therapy Aide

Where: Tampa, Florida

INSIDER'S STORY

I came to the United States from Barbados three years ago. In Barbados, I was an occupational therapist myself. I worked with physically handicapped children and teenagers. I moved here to be with my family (my wife is a dual citizen, and is studying law at a university here). Because the standards are different here, I don't have U.S. certification to work as an occupational therapist.

I work in the rehabilitative area of a retirement community. We also provide nursing and long-term care for terminally ill people or those who just can't take care of themselves any longer, but most of the people I work with are recovering from a stroke, accident or surgery, and do plan to return to their homes eventually. They are all elderly people—there's no shortage of jobs in nursing homes and retirement communities in this part of the country. I was raised by my grandparents, so I've always had a soft spot for older people. I think it's a great skill to take care of people in a way that is caring and respectful.

My responsibilities as an aide are more limited then they were as a therapist, but the goal of the therapy is the same: to help people restore the skills they need to go back to their everyday activities. For some people, that means learning to live with injuries or loss of movement and knowing how to do things in a new way. For others, it can mean something as simple as practicing tying their shoes. The work I do here is primarily administrative and organizational, coordinating the different functions of the clinic so that the therapists can concentrate on their work.

Patience is an extremely important part of working in occupational therapy. Most of the time, the skills and movements we work to restore are small things, things people don't even think about until they aren't able to do them anymore. It can seem mundane, but also gives you a new appreciation for your health. Watching someone struggle for an hour just to hold a spoon the right way—it makes you realize how much we take our bodies for granted.

I am working toward being certified as an occupational therapist in the United States. This position isn't the work I'm used to doing, but it's good for me to be making contacts in the OT field. It also gives me an opportunity to practice my English language skills. I hope to be able to use my training to pass an occupational therapist assistant certification exam, and at some point become a full therapist. My employer has been very supportive, and is even helping me to pay to take some of the classes I need. I'm optimistic about my future here, and I'm looking forward to working in this field for years to come.

Professional Associations and Accrediting Agencies

PROFESSIONAL ASSOCIATIONS

American Association of Homes and Services for the Aging
2519 Connecticut Avenue NW
Washington, DC 20008-1520
Phone: 202-783-2242
Fax: 202-783-2255
www.aahsa.org

American Association of Medical Assistants
20 N. Wacker Drive, #1575
Chicago, IL 60606-2963
Phone: 312-899-1500
www.aama-ntl.org

American Healthcare Radiology Administrators
111 Boston Post Road
Suite 105
Sudbury, MA 01776
Toll Free: 800-334-2472
Phone: 978-443-7591
Fax: 978-443-8046
www.ahraonline.org

American Health Information Management Association (*formerly American Medical Records Association*)
233 N. Michigan Avenue, Suite 2150
Chicago, IL 60601-5800
Phone: 312-233-1100
Fax: 312-233-1090
www.ahima.org

American Medical Technologists
710 Higgins Road
Park Ridge, IL
60068-5765
Phone: 847-823-5169
Fax: 847-823-0458
www.amt1.com

**The American Registry of Diagnostic
Medical Sonographers**

600 Jefferson Plaza, Suite 360

Rockville, MD 20852-1150

Phone: 301-738-8401 / 800-541-9754

Fax: 301-738-0312 / 301-738-0313

www.ardms.org

**The American Registry of Radiologic
Technologists**

1255 Northland Drive

St. Paul, MN 55120-1155

Phone 651-687-0048

www.arrt.org

**American Society of Podiatric
Medical Assistants**

Executive Office

2124 South Austin Blvd.

Cicero, IL 60804

Phone: 708-863-6303 / 1-888-88ASPMA

www.aspma.org

National Association for Home Care

228 7th Street SE

Washington, DC 20003

Phone: 202-547-7424

Fax: 202-547-3540

www.nahc.org

**National Health Occupations
Students of America**

6021 Morriss Road, Suite 111

Flower Mound, TX 75028

Phone: 800-321-HOSA

Fax: 972-874-0063

www.hosa.org

ACCREDITING BODIES FOR HEALTHCARE TRAINING PROGRAMS

**Accrediting Bureau of Health
Education Schools**

803 W. Broad Street, Suite 730

Falls Church, VA 22046

Phone: 703-533-2082

www.abhes.org

**Commission on Accreditation of
Allied Health Education Programs**

35 East Wacker Drive, Suite 1970

Chicago, IL 60601-2208

Phone 312-553-9355

Fax 312-553-9616

www.caahep.org

Joint Commission on Allied Health
Personnel in Ophthalmology

2025 Woodlane Drive

St. Paul, MN 55125-2995

Phone: 651-731-2944 or 888-284-3937

Fax: 651-731-0410

www.jcahpo.org

Joint Commission on Accreditation
of Healthcare Organizations

One Renaissance Boulevard

Oakbrook Terrace, IL 60181

Phone: 630-792-5000

Fax: 630-792-5005

www.jcaho.org

Joint Review Committee on
Education in Radiologic
Technology

20 N. Wacker Drive, Suite 900

Chicago, IL 60606-2901

Phone: 312-704-5300

Fax: 312-704-5304

www.jrcert.org

Liaison Council on Certification for
the Surgical Technologist

7790 East Arapahoe Road, Suite 240

Englewood, CO 80112-1274

Phone: 303-694-9264 / 800-707-0057

Fax: 303-689-0518

www.lcc-st.org

National Accrediting Agency for
Clinical Laboratory Sciences

8410 W Bryn Mawr Avenue, Suite 670

Chicago, IL 60631

Phone: 773-714-8880

Fax: 773-714-8886

www.naacls.org

NATIONAL ACCREDITING AGENCIES

Here is a list of national accrediting agencies for you to contact to see if your chosen school is accredited. You can request a list of schools that each agency accredits.

Accrediting Commission for Career Schools and Colleges of Technology (ACCSCT)
2101 Wilson Boulevard, Suite 302
Arlington, VA 22201
Phone: 703-247-4212
Fax: 703-247-4533
www.accsct.org

Accrediting Council for Independent Colleges and Schools (ACICS)
750 First Street NE, Suite 980
Washington, DC 20002-4241
Phone: 202-336-6780
Fax: 202-842-2593
www.acics.org

Distance Education and Training Council (DETC)
1601 Eighteenth Street NW
Washington, DC 20009-2529
Phone: 202-234-5100
Fax: 202-332-1386
www.detc.org

REGIONAL ACCREDITING AGENCIES

Middle States

New England States

Middle States Association of Colleges and Schools
Commission on Institutions of Higher Education
3624 Market Street
Philadelphia, PA 19104-2680
Phone: 215-662-5606
Fax: 215-662-5950
www.msache.org

New England Association of Schools and Colleges
Commission on Institutions of Higher Education (NEASC-CIHE)
209 Burlington Road
Bedford, MA 07130-1433
Phone: 781-271-0022 x313
Fax: 781-271-0950
www.neasc.org/cihe

New England Association of Schools and Colleges

Commission on Vocational, Technical and Career Institution (NEASC-CTCI)

209 Burlington Road

Bedford, MA 01730-1433

Phone: 781-271-0022 x316

Fax: 781-271-0950

www.neasc.org/ctci

North Central States

North Central Association of Colleges and Schools

Commission on Institutions of Higher Education (NCA)

30 North LaSalle, Suite 2400

Chicago, IL 60602-2504

Phone: 312-263-0456 / 800-621-7440

Fax: 312-263-7462

www.ncahihe.org

Northwest States

Northwest Association of Schools and Colleges

Commission on Colleges

11130 NE 33rd Place, Suite 120

Bellevue, WA 98004

Phone: 425-827-2005

Fax: 425-827-3395

www.cocnase.org

Southern States

Southern Association of Colleges and Schools

Commission on Colleges (SACS)

1866 Southern Lane

Decatur, GA 30033-4097

Phone: 404-679-4500 / 800-248-7701

Fax: 404-679-4558

www.sacscoc.org

Western States

Western Association of Schools and Colleges

Accrediting Commission for Community and Junior Colleges (WASC-Jr.)

3402 Mendocino Ave.

Santa Rosa, CA 95403-2244

Phone: 707-569-9177

Fax: 707-569-9179

www.accjc.org

Western Association of Schools and Colleges

Accrediting Commission for Senior Colleges and Universities (WASC-Sr.)

985 Atlantic Avenue, Suite 100

Alameda, CA 94501

Phone: 510-632-5000

Fax: 510-632-8361

www.wascsenior.org/senior/wascsr.html

FINANCIAL AID FROM STATE HIGHER EDUCATION AGENCIES

You can request information about financial aid from each of the following state higher education agencies and governing boards.

Alabama

**Alabama Commission on Higher
    Education**
100 North Union Street
P.O. Box 302000
Montgomery, AL 36130-2000
334-281-1998; fax 334-242-0268
www.ache.state.al.us

State Department of Education
50 North Ripley Street
P.O. Box 302101
Montgomery, AL 36104
205-242-8082
www.alsde.edu

Alaska

**Alaska Commission on
    Postsecondary Education**
3030 Vintage Boulevard
Juneau, AK 99801-7100
907-465-2962; 800-441-2962;
    fax 907-465-5316
www.state.ak.us/acpe

State Department of Education
801 West 10th Street, Suite 200
Juneau, AK 99801
907-465-2800; fax 907-465-3452
www.educ.state.ak.us

Arizona

Arizona Board of Regents
2020 N. Central Avenue, Suite 230
Phoenix, AZ 85004-4593
602-229-2500; fax 602-229-2555
www.abor.asu.edu

State Department of Education
1535 West Jefferson Street
Phoenix, AZ 85007
602-542-4361; 800-352-4558
www.ade.state.az.us

Arkansas

**Arkansas Department of Higher
    Education**
144 E. Capitol Avenue
Little Rock, AR 72201
501-371-2000
www.arkansashighered.com

Arkansas Department of Education
4 State Capitol Mall, Room 304A
Little Rock, AR 72201-1071
501-682-4474
arkedu.state.ar.us

California

California Student Aid Commission
P.O. Box 419027
Rancho Cordova, CA 95741-9027
916-445-0880; 888-224-7268;
    fax 916-526-8002
www.csac.ca.gov

California Department of Education
721 Capitol Mall
Sacramento, CA 95814
916-657-2451
goldmine.cde.ca.gov

Colorado

Colorado Commission on Higher Education
1380 Lawrence Street, Suite 1200
Denver, CO 80204
303-866-2723; fax 303-866-4266
www.state.co.us/cche_dir/hecche.html

State Department of Education
201 East Colfax Avenue
Denver, CO 80203-1799
303-866-6600; fax 303-830-0793
www.cde.state.co.us

Connecticut

Connecticut Department of Higher Education
61 Woodland Street
Hartford, CT 06105-2326
860-947-1800; fax 860-947-1310
www.ctdhe.org

Connecticut Department of Education
P.O. Box 2219
Hartford, CT 06145
860-566-5677
www.state.ct.us/sde

Delaware

Delaware Higher Education Commission
820 N. French Street
Wilmington, DE 19801
302-577-3240; 800-292-7935;
    fax 302-577-5765
www.doe.state.de.us/high-ed

District of Columbia

Department of Human Services
Office of Postsecondary Education,
    Research, and Assistance
2100 Martin Luther King Jr. Avenue SE,
    Suite 401
Washington, DC 20020
202-727-3685

District of Columbia Public Schools
Division of Student Services
4501 Lee Street NE
Washington, DC 20019
202-724-4934
www.k12.dc.us

Florida

Florida Department of Education
Turlington Building
325 West Gaines Street
Tallahassee, FL 32399-0400
904-487-0649
www.firn.edu/doe

Georgia

Georgia Student Finance
   Commission
State Loans and Grants Division
Suite 245, 2082 E. Exchange Place
Tucker, GA 30084
404-414-3000
www.gsfc.org

State Department of Education
2054 Twin Towers East, 205 Butler St.
Atlanta, GA 30334-5040
404-656-5812
www.glc.k12.state.ga.us

Hawaii

Hawaii Department of Education
2530 10th Avenue, Room A12
Honolulu, HI 96816
808-733-9103
www.doe.k12.hi.us

Idaho

Idaho Board of Education
P.O. Box 83720
Boise, ID 83720-0037
208-334-2270
www.sde.state.id.us/osbe/board.htm

State Department of Education
650 West State Street
Boise, ID 83720
208-332-6800
www.sde.state.id.us

Illinois

Illinois Student Assistance
   Commission
1755 Lake Cook Road
Deerfield, IL 60015-5209
708-948-8500
www.isac1.org

Indiana

**State Student Assistance
Commission of Indiana**
150 W. Market Street, Suite 500
Indianapolis, IN 46204-2811
317-232-2350; 888-528-4719;
    fax 317-232-3260
www.in.gov/ssaci

Indiana Department of Education
Room 229, State House
Indianapolis, IN 46204-2798
317-232-2305
ideanet.doe.state.in.us

Iowa

**Iowa College Student Aid
Commission**
200 10th Street, 4th Floor
Des Moines, IA 50309-2036
515-242-3344
www.state.ia.us/collegeaid

Iowa Department of Education
Grimes State Office Building
Des Moines, IA 50319-0146
515-281-5294; fax 515-242-5988
www.state.ia.us/educate

Kansas

Kansas Board of Regents
1000 SW Jackson Street, Suite 520
Topeka, KS 66612-1368785-296-3421
www.kansasregents.org

State Department of Education
Kansas State Education Bldg.
120 E. Tenth Avenue
Topeka, KS 66612-1103
785-296-3201; fax 785-296-7933
www.ksbe.state.ks.us

Kentucky

**Kentucky Higher Education
Assistance Authority**
Suite 102, 1050 U.S. 127 South
Frankfort, KY 40601-4323
800-928-8926
www.kheaa.com

State Department of Education
500 Mero Street
Frankfort, KY 40601
502-564-4770; 800-533-5372
www.kde.state.ky.us

Louisiana

Louisiana Student Financial Assistance Commission
Office of Student Financial Assistance
P.O. Box 91202
Baton Rouge, LA 70821-9202
800-259-5626
www.osfa.state.la.us

State Department of Education
P.O. Box 94064
626 North 4th Street, 12th Floor
Baton Rouge, LA 70804-9064
504-342-2098; 877-453-2721
www.doe.state.la.us

Maine

Finance Authority of Maine
5 Community Drive
P.O. Box 949
Augusta, ME 04333-0949
207-287-3263; 800-228-3734;
    fax 207- 623-0095
www.famemaine.com/html/education

Maine Department of Education
23 State House Station
Augusta, ME 04333-0023
207-287-5800; fax 207-287-5900
www.state.me.us/education

Maryland

Maryland Higher Education Commission
Jeffrey Building, 16 Francis St.
Annapolis, MD 21401-1781
410-974-2971
www.mhec.state.md.us

Maryland State Department of Education
200 West Baltimore Street
Baltimore, MD 21201-2595
410-767-0100
www.msde.state.md.us

Massachusetts

Massachusetts Board of Higher Education
One Ashburton Place, Room 1401
Boston, MA 02108
617-727-9420
www.mass.edu

State Department of Education
350 Main Street
Malden, MA 02148-5023
781-338-3300
www.doe.mass.edu

Massachusetts Higher Education Information Center
700 Boylston Street
Boston, MA 02116
617-536-0200; 877-332-4348
www.heic.org

Michigan

Michigan Higher Education Assistance Authority

Office of Scholarships and Grants

P.O. Box 30462

Lansing, MI 48909-7962

517-373-3394; 877-323-2287

www.mi-studentaid.org

Michigan Department of Education

608 W. Allegan Street, Hannah Building

Lansing, MI 48909

517-373-3324

www.mde.state.mi.us

Minnesota

Minnesota Higher Education Services Office

1450 Energy Park Drive, Suite 350

Saint Paul, MN 55108-5227

651-642-0533; 800-657-3866;

    fax 651-642-0675

www.mheso.state.mn.us

Department of Children, Families, and Learning

1500 Highway 36 West

Roseville, MN 55113

651-582-8200

www.educ.state.mn.us

Mississippi

Mississippi Postsecondary Education

Financial Assistance Board

3825 Ridgewood Road

Jackson, MS 39211-6453

601-982-6663

State Department of Education

Central High School, P.O. Box 771

359 North West Street

Jackson, MS 39205-0771

601-359-3513

www.mde.k12.ms.us

Missouri

Missouri Coordinating Board for Higher Education

3515 Amazonas Drive

Jefferson City, MO 65109-5717

314-751-2361; 800-473-6757;

    fax 573-751-6635

www.cbhe.state.mo.us

Missouri State Department of Elementary and Secondary Education

P.O. Box 480

Jefferson City, MO 65102-0480

573-751-4212; fax 573-751-8613

www.dese.state.mo.us

Montana

Montana Higher Education Student Assistance Corporation

2500 Broadway

Helena, MT 59620-3104

406-444-6597; 1-800-852-2761 x 0606;
   fax 406-444-0684

www.mhesac.org

Montana Office of the Commissioner of Higher Education

2500 Broadway

P.O. Box 203101

Helena, MT 59620-3101

406-444-6570; fax 406-444-1469

www.montana.edu/wwwoche

State Office of Public Instruction

P.O. Box 202501

Helena, MT 59620-2501

406-444-3680; 888-231-9393

www.metnet.state.mt.us

Nebraska

Coordinating Commission for Postsecondary Education

P.O. Box 95005

Lincoln, NE 68509-5005

402-471-2847; fax 402-471-2886

www.ccpe.state.ne.us

Nebraska Department of Education

301 Centennial Mall South

Lincoln, NE 68509-4987

402-471-2295

www.nde.state.ne.us

Nevada

Nevada Department of Education

700 East Fifth Street

Carson City, NV 89701-5096

775-687-9200; fax 775-687-9101

www.nde.state.nv.us

New Hampshire

New Hampshire Postsecondary Education Commission

2 Industrial Park Drive

Concord, NH 03301-8512

603-271-2555; fax 603-271-2696

www.state.nh.us/postsecondary

State Department of Education

State Office Park South

101 Pleasant Street

Concord, NH 03301

603-271-3494; fax 603-271-1953

www.state.nh.us/doe

New Jersey

State of New Jersey
20 West State Street
P.O. Box 542
Trenton, NJ 08625-0542
609-292-4310;
fax 609-292-7225; 800-792-8670
www.state.nj.us/highereducation

State Department of Education
225 West State Street
Trenton, NJ 08625-0500
609-984-6409
www.state.nj.us/education

New Mexico

New Mexico Commission on Higher Education
1068 Cerrillos Road
Santa Fe, NM 87501-4925
505-827-7383; fax 505-827-7392
www.nmche.org

State Department of Education
Education Building
300 Don Gaspar
Santa Fe, NM 87501-2786
505-827-6648
www.sde.state.nm.us

New York

New York State Higher Education Services Corporation
One Commerce Plaza
Albany, NY 12255
518-473-1574; 888-697-4372
www.hesc.state.ny.us

State Education Department
89 Washington Avenue
Albany, NY 12234
518-474-3852
www.nysed.gov

North Carolina

North Carolina State Education Assistance Authority
P.O. Box 14103
Research Triangle Park, NC 27709
919-549-8614; fax 919-549-8481
www.ncseaa.edu

State Department of Public Instruction
301 N. Wilmington Street
Raleigh, NC 27601
919-807-3300
www.dpi.state.nc.us

North Dakota

North Dakota University System/State Board of Higher Education
10th Floor, State Capitol
600 East Boulevard Ave, Dept. 215
Bismarck, ND 58505-0230
701-328-2960; fax 701-328-2961
www.ndus.edu/sbhe

State Department of Public Instruction
State Capitol Bldg., 11th Floor
600 E. Boulevard Avenue, Dept. 201
Bismarck, ND 58505-0164
701-328-2260; fax 701-328-2461
www.dpi.state.nd.us

Ohio

State Department of Education
25 South Front Street
Columbus, OH 43266-0308
614-466-2761; 877-644-6338
www.ode.state.oh.us

Oklahoma

Oklahoma State Regents for Higher Education
655 Research Parkway, Suite 200
Oklahoma City, OK 73104
405-225-9100; fax 405-225-9230
www.okhighered.org

Oklahoma Guaranteed Student Loan Program
P.O. Box 3000
Oklahoma City, OK 73101-3000
405-858-4300;
fax 405-234-4390; 800-247-0420
www.ogslp.org

State Department of Education
Oliver Hodge Memorial Education Building
2500 North Lincoln Boulevard
Oklahoma City, OK 73105-4599
405-521-4122; fax 405-521-6205
www.sde.state.ok.us

Oregon

Oregon Student Assistance Commission
Suite 100, 1500 Valley River Drive
Eugene, OR 97401-2130
503-687-7400
www.osac.state.or.us

Oregon State System of Higher Education
P.O. Box 3175
Eugene, OR 97403
541-346-5700
www.ous.edu

Oregon Department of Education
255 Capitol St. NE
Salem, OR 97310-0203
503-378-3569; fax 503-378-2892
www.ode.state.or.us

Pennsylvania

Pennsylvania Higher Education Assistance Agency
1200 North Seventh Street
Harrisburg, PA 17102-1444
800-692-7392
www.pheaa.org

Rhode Island

Rhode Island Office of Higher Education
301 Promenade Street
Providence, RI 02908-5748
401-222-2088; fax 401-222-2545
www.ribghe.org

Rhode Island Higher Education Assistance Authority
560 Jefferson Boulevard
Warwick, RI 02886
800-922-9855; fax 401-736-1100
www.riheaa.org

State Department of Education
225 Westminster Street
Providence, RI 02903
401-222-4600
www.ridoe.net

South Carolina

South Carolina Higher Education Tuition Grants Commission
101 Business Park Boulevard, Suite 2100
Columbia, SC 29203-9498
803-896-1120; fax 803-896-1126
www.sctuitiongrants.com

State Department of Education
1429 Senate Street
Columbia, SC 29201
803-734-8500
www.sde.state.sc.us

South Dakota

Department of Education and Cultural Affairs
700 Governors Drive
Pierre, SD 57501-2291
605-773-3134
www.state.sd.us/deca

South Dakota Board of Regents
306 East Capitol Ave., Suite 200
Pierre, SD 57501-2409
605-773-3455
www.ris.sdbor.edu

Tennessee

Tennessee Higher Education Commission
404 James Robertson Parkway, Suite 1900
Nashville, TN 37243-0820
615-741-3605; fax 615-741-6230
www.state.tn.us/thec

State Department of Education
6th Floor, Andrew Johnson Tower
710 James Robertson Parkway
Nashville, TN 37243-0375
615-741-2731
www.state.tn.us/education

Texas

Texas Education Agency
1701 North Congress Avenue
Austin, TX 78701-1494512- 463-9734
www.tea.state.tx.us

Texas Higher Education Coordinating Board
P.O. Box 12788
Austin, TX 78711
512-427-6101; 800-242-3062
www.thecb.state.tx.us

Utah

Utah System of Higher Education
#3 Triad Center, Suite 550
Salt Lake City, UT 84180-1205
801-321-7101
www.utahsbr.edu

Utah State Office of Education
250 East 500 South
Salt Lake City, UT 84111
801-538-7500; fax 801-538-7521
www.usoe.k12.ut.us

Vermont

Vermont Student Assistance Corporation
Champlain Mill
P.O. Box 2000
Winooski, VT 05404-2601
802-655-9602; 800-642-3177;
fax 802-654-3765
www.vsac.org

Vermont Department of Education
120 State Street
Montpelier, VT 05620-2501
802-828-3147; fax 802-828-3140
www.state.vt.us/educ

Virginia

State Council of Higher Education for Virginia
James Monroe Building, 101 N. 14th Street
Richmond, VA 23219
804-225-2628; fax 804 225-2638
www.schev.edu

State Department of Education
P.O. Box 2120
Richmond, VA 23218-2120
800-292-3820
www.pen.k12.va.us

West Virginia

State Department of Education
1900 Kanawha Boulevard East
Charleston, WV 25305
304-558-2691
wvde.state.wv.us

State College and University Systems of West Virginia Central Office
1018 Kanawha Boulevard East, Suite 700
Charleston, WV 25301-2827
304-558-2101; fax 304-558-5719
www.hepc.wvnet.edu

Washington

Washington State Higher Education Coordinating Board
P.O. Box 43430, 917 Lakeridge Way, SW
Olympia, WA 98504-3430
206-753-7800
www.hecb.wa.gov

State Department of Public Instruction
Old Capitol Building, P.O. Box 47200
Olympia, WA 98504-7200
360-725-6000
www.k12.wa.us

Wisconsin

Higher Educational Aids Board
P.O. Box 7885
Madison, WI 53707-7885
608-267-2206; fax 608-267-2808
www.heab.state.wi.us

State Department of Public Instruction
125 South Webster Street
P.O. Box 7841
Madison, WI 53707-7814
608-266-3390; 800-541-4563
www.dpi.state.wi.us

Wyoming

Wyoming State Department of Education
Hathaway Bldg., 2300 Capitol Avenue, 2nd Floor
Cheyenne, WY 82002-0050
307-777-7675; fax 307-777-6234
www.k12.wy.us/wdehome.html

Wyoming Community College Commission
2020 Carey Avenue, 8th Floor
Cheyenne, WY 82002
307-777-7763; fax 307-777-6567
www.commission.wcc.edu

Puerto Rico

Council on Higher Education
P.O. Box 19900
San Juan, PR 00910-1900
787-724-7100
www.ces.gobierno.pr

Department of Education
P. O. Box 190759
San Juan, PR 00919-0759
809-759-2000; fax 809-250-0275

U.S. Department of Education

Students.gov (Students' Gateway to the U.S. Government)
400 Maryland Avenue SW
ROB-3, Room 4004
Washington, DC 20202-5132
www.students.gov

U.S. Department of Education
Office of Postsecondary Education
1990 K Street NW
Washington, DC 20006
www.ed.gov/offices/OPE

Additional Resources

For additional information on the topics discussed in this book, refer to the following reading lists, which are organized by subject.

BUSINESS WRITING

Bartell, Karen H. *American Business English*. Ann Arbor: University of Michigan, 1995.

Chesla, Elizabeth. *Improve Your Writing for Work*. New York: LearningExpress, 1997.

Heller, Bernard. *The 100 Most Difficult Business Letters You'll Ever Have to Write, Fax, or E-Mail*. New York: HarperBusiness, 1994.

Piotrwoski, Maryann V. *Effective Business Writing: A Guide for Those Who Write on the Job*. New York: HarperCollins, 1996.

Stuckey, Marty. *Basics of Business Writing (Worksmart Series)*. New York: Amacom, 1992.

Venolia, Jan. *Better Letters: A Handbook of Business and Personal Correspondence*. Berkeley, CA: Ten Speed Press, 1995.

COLLEGES

Chronicle Vocational School Manual: A Directory of Accredited Vocational and Technical Schools 2000–2001. Moravia, NY: Chronicle Guidance, 2000.

The College Board. *The College Handbook* (annual). New York: College Entrance Examination Board.

Peterson's Guide to Distance Learning Programs (annual). Princeton, NJ: Peterson's.

Peterson's Guide to Two-Year Colleges (annual). Princeton, NJ: Peterson's.

COVER LETTERS

Beatty, Richard H. *The Perfect Cover Letter.* 2nd Ed. New York: John Wiley & Sons, 1997.

Besson, Taunee. *The Wall Street Journal National Business Employment Weekly: Cover Letters.* 3rd Ed. New York: John Wiley & Sons, 1999.

Enelow, Wendy and Louise Kursmark. *Cover Letter Magic.* Indianapolis: Jist Works, 2000.

Marler, Patty and Jan Bailey Mattia. *Cover Letters Made Easy.* Lincolnwood, IL: NTC Publishing Group, 1995.

Yates, Martin. *Cover Letters That Knock'Em Dead.* Holbrook, MA: Adams Media Corp., 2000.

FINANCIAL AID

Cassidy, Daniel. *Last Minute College Financing.* Franklin Lakes, NJ: Career Press, 2000.

College Board. *College Costs & Financial Aid Handbook 1999.* 19th Ed. New York: College Entrance Examination Board, 1998.

Finney, David F. *Financing Your College Degree: A Guide for Adult Students.* New York: College Entrance Examination Board, 1997.

HEALTHCARE CAREER RESOURCES

Fox-Rose, Joan. *Opportunities in Nursing Assistant Careers.* New York: McGraw-Hill/NTC, 1999.

McMahon, Christine. *Care of the Older Person: A Handbook for Care Assistants.* Oxford: Blackwell Science, 1997.

Metcalf, Zubie. *Career Planning Guide for the Allied Health Professions*. New York: Lippincott, Williams & Wilkins, 1997.

Quinlan, Kathryn A. *Physical Therapist Assistant (Careers Without College series)*. Mankato, MN: Capstone Press, 1998.

Roberts, Ellen C. *The Home Care Aide's Quick Reference Guide*. New York: Prentice Hall, 1999.

VGM Career. *Resumes for Health and Medical Careers*. New York: McGraw-Hill/NTC, 1997.

Weiss, Roberta. *Physical Therapy Aide*. Albany, NY: Delmar, 1998.

Zucker, Elana. *The Homemaker/Home Health Aide Pocket Guide*. New York: Prentice Hall, 2001.

INTERNSHIPS

Anselmi, John et al. *The Yale Daily News Guide to Internships* (annual). New York: Kaplan.

Hamadeh, Samer and Mark Oldham. *America's Top Internships* (annual). New York: Random House, The Princeton Review.

INTERVIEWS

Bloch, Deborah. *How to Have A Winning Interview*. Lincolnwood, IL: VGM Career Horizons, 1998.

Eyre, Vivian, et al. *Great Interview: Successful Strategies for Getting Hired*. New York: LearningExpress, 2000.

Fry, Ron. *101 Great Answers to the Toughest Interview Questions*. Franklin Lakes, NJ: Career Press, 2000.

Medley, H. Anthony. *Sweaty Palms: The Neglected Art of Being Interviewed*. Berkeley, CA: Ten Speed Press, 1992.

JOB HUNTING

For a listing of job search websites, see page 108 (Chapter 4).

U.S. Department of Labor. *Occupational Outlook Handbook* (annual). Lincolnwood, IL: NTC Publishing Group.

Bolles, Richard Nelson. *What Color Is Your Parachute? 2001: A Practical Manual for Job-Hunters and Career-Changers*. Berkeley: Ten Speed Press, 2000.

Cubbage, Sue and Marcia Williams. *National Job Hotline Directory: The Job Finder's Hot List*. River Forest, IL: Planning/Communications, 1998.

PERIODICALS

*Advance for Physical Therapists and PT
   Assistants*
2900 Horizon Drive
King of Prussia, PA 19406
www.advanceforpt.com

Caregiving . . . for Professionals Newsletter
Tad Publishing Co.
P.O. Box 224
Park Ridge, IL 60068
www.caregiving.com

Caring Magazine
228 Seventh Street SE
Washington, DC 20003
www.caringmagazine.com

Home Health Aide Digest
nuCompass Publishing
2724 9th Street
East Glencoe, MN 55336
www.hhadigest.com

Professional Medical Assistant
American Association of Medical Assistants
Attn: Magazine Subscriptions
20 N. Wacker Drive, Suite 1575
Chicago, IL 60606-2903
www.aama-ntl.org./pma/pma.html

RESUMES

Rich, Jason R. *Great Resume: Get Noticed, Get Hired.* New York: Learning Express, 2000.

Whitcomb, Susan. *Resume Magic: Trade Secrets of a Professional Resume Writer.* Indianapolis: Jist Works, 1998.

Yates, Martin. *Resumes That Knock 'Em Dead.* Holbrook, MA: Adams Media Corp., 2000.

SCHOLARSHIP GUIDES

Cassidy, Daniel J. *The Scholarship Book: The Complete Guide to Private-Sector Scholarships, Fellowships, Grants, and Loans for the Undergraduate* (annual). New York: Prentice Hall.

Fenner, Susan, et al. *Complete Office Handbook: The Definitive Resource for Today's Electronic Office.* New York: Random House, 1996.

Kaplan, Benjamin. *How to Go to College Almost for Free: The Secrets of Winning Scholarship Money.* New York: Harper Resource, 2001.

McKee, Cynthia Ruiz and Philip McKee. *Cash for College: The Ultimate Guide to College Scholarships.* New York: Quill, 1999.

Ragins, Marianne. *Winning Scholarships for College: An Insider's Guide.* New York: Henry Holt, 1999.

STUDYING

Chesla, Elizabeth. *Read Better, Remember More* (Basics Made Easy series). 2nd edition. New York: LearningExpress, 2000.

Wood, Gail. *How to Study* (Basics Made Easy series). 2nd edition. New York: Learning Express, 2000.

TEST HELP

Ehrenhaft, George, et al. *Barron's How to Prepare for the SAT: American College Testing Assessment*. 12th Ed. New York: Barron's Educational, 2001.

Robinson, Adam, et al. *Cracking the SAT & PSAT* (annual). Princeton, NJ: Princeton Review.

Appendix C

Sample Free Application for Federal Student Aid (FAFSA)

On the following pages you will find a sample FAFSA. Use this form to familiarize yourself with the form so that when you apply for federal and state student grants, work-study, and loans, you will know what information you need to have ready. At print this was the most current form available, and although the form remains mostly the same from year to year, you should check the FAFSA website (www.fafsa.ed.gov) for the most current information.

2001-2002

The **FAFSA**

July 1, 2001 — June 30, 2002
Free Application for Federal Student Aid

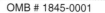

OMB # 1845-0001

Use this form to apply for federal and state* student grants, work-study, and loans.

Apply over the Internet with 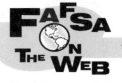 **www.fafsa.ed.gov**

If you are filing a **2000 income tax return,** we recommend that you complete it before filling out this form. However, you do not need to file your income tax return with the IRS before you submit this form.

If you or your family has **unusual circumstances** (such as loss of employment) that might affect your need for student financial aid, submit this form, and then consult with the financial aid office at the college you plan to attend.

You may also use this form to apply for **aid from other sources, such as your state or college.** The deadlines for states (see table to right) or colleges may be as early as January 2001 and may differ. You may be required to complete additional forms. Check with your high school guidance counselor or a financial aid administrator at your college about state and college sources of student aid.

Your answers on this form will be read electronically. Therefore:

- use black ink and fill in ovals completely:
- print clearly in CAPITAL letters and skip a box between words:
- report dollar amounts (such as $12,356.41) like this:

Yes ●   No ✗ ✓

| I | 5 | | E | L | M | | S | T |

$ | | 1 | 2 | , | 3 | 5 | 6 | **no cents**

Green is for students and purple is for parents.

If you have questions about this application, or for more information on eligibility requirements and the U.S. Department of Education's student aid programs, look on the Internet at **www.ed.gov/studentaid** You can also call 1-800-4FED-AID (1-800-433-3243) seven days a week from 8:00 a.m. through midnight (Eastern time). TTY users may call 1-800-730-8913.

After you complete this application, make a copy of it for your records. Then **send the original of pages 3 through 6** in the attached envelope or send it to: Federal Student Aid Programs, P.O. Box 4008, Mt. Vernon, IL 62864-8608.

You should submit your application as early as possible, but no earlier than January 1, 2001. We must receive your application **no later than July 1, 2002.** Your school must have your correct, complete information by your last day of enrollment in the 2001-2002 school year.

You should hear from us within four weeks. If you do not, please call 1-800-433-3243 or check on-line at www.fafsa.ed.gov

Now go to page 3 and begin filling out this form.
Refer to the notes as needed.

STATE AID DEADLINES

AR April 1, 2001 *(date received)*
AZ June 30, 2002 *(date received)*
*^ CA March 2, 2001 *(date postmarked)*
* DC June 24, 2001 *(date received by state)*
DE April 15, 2001 *(date received)*
FL May 15, 2001 *(date processed)*
HI March 1, 2001
^ IA July 1, 2001 *(date received)*
IL First-time applicants – September 30, 2001
    Continuing applicants – July 15, 2001
    (date received)
^ IN For priority consideration – March 1, 2001
    (date postmarked)
* KS For priority consideration – April 1, 2001
    (date received)
KY For priority consideration – March 15, 2001
    (date received)
^ LA For priority consideration – April 15, 2001
    Final deadline – July 1, 2001
    (date received)
^ MA For priority consideration – May 1, 2001
    (date received)
MD March 1, 2001 *(date postmarked)*
ME May 1, 2001 *(date received)*
MI High school seniors – February 21, 2001
    College students – March 21, 2001
    (date received)
MN June 30, 2002 *(date received)*
MO April 1, 2001 *(date received)*
MT For priority consideration – March 1, 2001
    (date postmarked)
NC March 15, 2001 *(date received)*
ND April 15, 2001 *(date processed)*
NH May 1, 2001 *(date received)*
^ NJ June 1, 2001 if you received a
    Tuition Aid Grant in 2000-2001
    All other applicants
    – October 1, 2001, for fall and spring term
    – March 1, 2002, for spring term only
    (date received)
*^ NY May 1, 2002 *(date postmarked)*
OH October 1, 2001 *(date received)*
OK For priority consideration – April 30, 2001
    Final deadline – June 30, 2001
    (date received)
OR May 1, 2002 *(date received)*
* PA All 2000-2001 State Grant recipients and
    non-2000-2001 State Grant recipients
    degree programs – May 1, 2001
    All other applicants – August 1, 2001
    (date received)
PR May 2, 2002 *(date application signed)*
RI March 1, 2001 *(date received)*
SC June 30, 2001 *(date received)*
TN May 1, 2001 *(date processed)*
*^ WV March 1, 2001 *(date received)*

Check with your financial aid administrator for these states: AK, AL, *AS, *CT, CO, *FM, GA, *GU, *HI, *MH, *MP, MS, *NE, *NM, *NV, *PW, *SD, *TX, UT, *VA, *VI, *VT, WA, WI, and *WY.

^ Applicants encouraged to obtain proof of mailing

* Additional form may be required

Notes for questions **13–14** (page 3)

If you are an eligible noncitizen, write in your eight or nine digit Alien Registration Number. Generally, you are an eligible noncitizen if you are: (1) a U.S. permanent resident and you have an Alien Registration Receipt Card (I-551); (2) a conditional permanent resident (I-551C); or (3) an other eligible noncitizen with an Arrival-Departure Record (I-94) from the U.S. Immigration and Naturalization Service showing any one of the following designations: "Refugee," "Asylum Granted," "Indefinite Parole," "Humanitarian Parole," or "Cuban-Haitian Entrant." If you are in the U.S. on only an F1 or F2 student visa, or only a J1 or J2 exchange visitor visa, or a G series visa (pertaining to international organizations), you must fill in oval **c**. If you are neither a citizen nor eligible noncitizen, you are not eligible for federal student aid. However, you may be eligible for state or college aid.

Notes for questions **17–21** (page 3)

For undergraduates, full time generally means taking at least 12 credit hours in a term or 24 clock hours per week. 3/4 time generally means taking at least 9 credit hours in a term or 18 clock hours per week. Half time generally means taking at least 6 credit hours in a term or 12 clock hours per week. Provide this information about the college you plan to attend.

Notes for question **29** (page 3) — Enter the correct number in the box in question 29.

Enter **1** for 1st bachelor's degree
Enter **2** for 2nd bachelor's degree
Enter **3** for associate degree (occupational or technical program)
Enter **4** for associate degree (general education or transfer program)
Enter **5** for certificate or diploma for completing an occupational, technical, or educational program of less than two years

Enter **6** for certificate or diploma for completing an occupational, technical, or educational program of at least two years
Enter **7** for teaching credential program (nondegree program)
Enter **8** for graduate or professional degree
Enter **9** for other/undecided

Notes for question **30** (page 3) — Enter the correct number in the box in question 30.

Enter **0** for 1st year undergraduate/never attended college
Enter **1** for 1st year undergraduate/attended college before
Enter **2** for 2nd year undergraduate/sophomore
Enter **3** for 3rd year undergraduate/junior

Enter **4** for 4th year undergraduate/senior
Enter **5** for 5th year/other undergraduate
Enter **6** for 1st year graduate/professional
Enter **7** for continuing graduate/professional or beyond

Notes for questions **37 c. and d.** (page 4) and **71 c. and d.** (page 5)

If you filed or will file a foreign tax return, or a tax return with Puerto Rico, Guam, American Samoa, the Virgin Islands, the Marshall Islands, the Federated States of Micronesia, or Palau, use the information from that return to fill out this form. If you filed a foreign return, convert all figures to U.S. dollars, using the exchange rate that is in effect today.

Notes for questions **38** (page 4) and **72** (page 5)

In general, a person is eligible to file a 1040A or 1040EZ if he or she makes less than $50,000, does not itemize deductions, does not receive income from his or her own business or farm, and does not receive alimony. A person is not eligible if he or she itemizes deductions, receives self-employment income or alimony, or is required to file Schedule D for capital gains.

Notes for questions **41** (page 4) and **75** (page 5) — only for people who filed a 1040EZ or Telefile

On the 1040EZ, if a person answered "Yes" on line 5, use EZ worksheet line F to determine the number of exemptions ($2,800 equals one exemption). If a person answered "No" on line 5, enter 01 if he or she is single, or 02 if he or she is married.

On the Telefile, use line J to determine the number of exemptions ($2,800 equals one exemption).

Notes for questions **47–48** (page 4) and **81–82** (page 5)

Net worth means current value minus debt. If net worth is one million or more, enter $999,999. If net worth is negative, enter 0.

Investments include real estate (do not include the home you live in), trust funds, money market funds, mutual funds, certificates of deposit, stocks, stock options, bonds, other securities, education IRAs, installment and land sale contracts (including mortgages held), commodities, etc. Investment value includes the market value of these investments as of today. Investment debt means only those debts that are related to the investments.

Investments do not include the home you live in, cash, savings, checking accounts, the value of life insurance and retirement plans (pension funds, annuities, noneducation IRAs, Keogh plans, etc.), or the value of prepaid tuition plans.

Business and/or investment farm value includes the market value of land, buildings, machinery, equipment, inventory, etc. Business and/or investment farm debt means only those debts for which the business or investment farm was used as collateral.

Notes for question **58** (page 4)

Answer **"No"** (you are not a veteran) if you (1) have never engaged in active duty in the U.S. Armed Forces, (2) are currently an ROTC student or a cadet or midshipman at a service academy, or (3) are a National Guard or Reserves enlistee activated only for training. Also answer "No" if you are currently serving in the U.S. Armed Forces and will continue to serve through June 30, 2002.

Answer **"Yes"** (you are a veteran) if you (1) have engaged in active duty in the U.S. Armed Forces (Army, Navy, Air Force, Marines, or Coast Guard) or as a member of the National Guard or Reserves who was called to active duty for purposes other than training, or were a cadet or midshipman at one of the service academies, **and** (2) were released under a condition other than dishonorable. Also answer "Yes" if you are not a veteran now but will be one by June 30, 2002.

The 2001-2002 FAFSA

Free Application for Federal Student Aid
For July 1, 2001 — June 30, 2002

OMB # 1845-0001

Step One: For questions 1-34, leave blank any questions that do not apply to you (the student).

1-3. Your full name (as it appears on your Social Security Card)

1. LAST NAME	2. FIRST NAME	3. MIDDLE INITIAL
FOR INFORMATION ONLY	DO NOT SUBMIT	

4-7. Your permanent mailing address

4. NUMBER AND STREET (INCLUDE APT. NUMBER)

5. CITY (AND COUNTRY IF NOT U.S.)   6. STATE   7. ZIP CODE

8. Your Social Security Number

XXX – XX – XXXX

9. Your date of birth

/ / 1 9

10. Your permanent telephone number

( ) –

11-12. Your driver's license number and state (if any)

11. LICENSE NUMBER   12. STATE

13. Are you a U.S. citizen? Pick one. **See Page 2.**

a. Yes, I am a U.S. citizen. .... ○ 1
b. No, but I am an eligible noncitizen. **Fill in question 14.** ...... ○ 2
c. No, I am not a citizen or eligible noncitizen. .... ○ 3

14. ALIEN REGISTRATION NUMBER

A

15. What is your marital status as of today?

I am single, divorced, or widowed. ○ 1
I am married/remarried. ○ 2
I am separated. ○ 3

16. Month and year you were married, separated, divorced, or widowed

MONTH / YEAR

For each question (17 - 21), please mark whether you will be full time, 3/4 time, half time, less than half time, or not attending. **See page 2.**

		Full time/Not sure	3/4 time	Half time	Less than half time	Not attending
17.	Summer 2001	○ 1	○ 2	○ 3	○ 4	○
18.	Fall 2001	○ 1	○ 2	○ 3	○ 4	○
19.	Winter 2001-2002	○ 1	○ 2	○ 3	○ 4	○
20.	Spring 2002	○ 1	○ 2	○ 3	○ 4	○
21.	Summer 2002	○ 1	○ 2	○ 3	○ 4	○

22. Highest school your father completed — Middle school/Jr. High ○ 1   High school ○ 2   College or beyond ○ 3   Other/unknown ○

23. Highest school your mother completed — Middle school/Jr. High ○ 1   High school ○ 2   College or beyond ○ 3   Other/unknown ○

24. What is your state of legal residence?   STATE

25. Did you become a legal resident of this state before January 1, 1996?   Yes ○ 1   No ○

26. If the answer to question 25 is **"No,"** give month and year you became a legal resident.   MONTH / YEAR

27. Are you male? (Most male students must register with Selective Service to get federal aid.)   Yes ○ 1   No ○

28. If you are male (age 18-25) and not registered, do you want Selective Service to register you?   Yes ○ 1   No ○

29. What degree or certificate will you be working on during 2001-2002? **See page 2** and enter the correct number in the box.

30. What will be your grade level when you begin the 2001-2002 school year? **See page 2** and enter the correct number in the box.

31. Will you have a high school diploma or GED before you enroll?   Yes ○ 1   No ○

32. Will you have your first bachelor's degree before July 1, 2001?   Yes ○ 1   No ○

33. In addition to grants, are you interested in student loans (which you must pay back)?   Yes ○ 1   No ○

34. In addition to grants, are you interested in "work-study" (which you earn through work)?   Yes ○ 1   No ○

35. Do not leave this question blank. Have you ever been convicted of possessing or selling illegal drugs? If you have, answer "Yes," complete and submit this application, and we will send you a worksheet in the mail for you to determine if your conviction affects your eligibility for aid.   No ○ 1   Yes ○ 3   DO NOT LEAVE QUESTION 35 BLANK

Step Two: For questions 36-49, report your (the student's) income and assets. If you are married, report your spouse's income and assets, even if you were not married in 2000. Ignore references to "spouse" if you are currently single, separated, divorced, or widowed.

36. For 2000, have you (the student) completed your IRS income tax return or another tax return listed in **question 37**?

   a. I have already completed my return. ○ 1   **b.** I will file, but I have not yet ○ 2   **c.** I'm not going to file. **(Skip to question 42.)** ○ 3
                                                      completed my return.

37. What income tax return did you file or will you file for 2000?

   a. IRS 1040 .... ○ 1   **d.** A tax return for Puerto Rico, Guam, American Samoa, the Virgin Islands, the
   b. IRS 1040A, 1040EZ, 1040Telefile ...... ○ 2   Marshall Islands, the Federated States of Micronesia, or Palau. **See Page 2.** ...... ○ 4
   c. A foreign tax return. **See Page 2.** ...... ○ 3

38. If you have filed or will file a 1040, were you eligible to file a 1040A or 1040EZ? **See page 2.**   **Yes** ○ 1 **No** ○ 2 **Don't Know** ○ 3

For questions 39-51, if the answer is zero or the question does not apply to you, enter 0.

39. What was your (and spouse's) adjusted gross income for 2000? Adjusted gross income is on IRS Form 1040–line 33; 1040A–line 19; 1040EZ–line 4; or Telefile–line I. $ [ ] , [ ]

40. Enter the total amount of your (and spouse's) income tax for 2000. Income tax amount is on IRS Form 1040–line 51; 1040A–line 33; 1040EZ–line 10; or Telefile–line K. $ [ ] , [ ]

41. Enter your (and spouse's) exemptions for 2000. Exemptions are on IRS Form 1040–line 6d or on Form 1040A–line 6d. For Form 1040EZ or Telefile, **see page 2.**   [ ]

42-43. How much did you (and spouse) earn from working in 2000? Answer this question whether or not you filed a tax return. This information may be on your W-2 forms, or on IRS Form 1040–lines 7 + 12 + 18; 1040A–line 7; or 1040EZ–line 1. Telefilers should use their W-2's.
   You (42) $ [ ] , [ ]
   Your Spouse (43) $ [ ] , [ ]

Student (and Spouse) Worksheets (44-46)

44-46. Go to Page 8 and complete the columns on the left of Worksheets A, B, and C. Enter the student (and spouse) totals in questions 44, 45, and 46, respectively. Even though you may have few of the Worksheet items, check each line carefully.
   Worksheet A (44) $ [ ] , [ ]
   Worksheet B (45) $ [ ] , [ ]
   Worksheet C (46) $ [ ] , [ ]

47. As of today, what is the net worth of your (and spouse's) current **investments**? **See page 2.** $ [ ] , [ ]

48. As of today, what is the net worth of your (and spouse's) current **businesses and/or investment farms**? **See page 2.** Do not include a farm that you live on and operate. $ [ ] , [ ]

49. As of today, what is your (and spouse's) total current balance of cash, savings, and checking accounts? $ [ ] , [ ]

50-51. If you receive veterans education benefits, for **how many months** from July 1, 2001 through June 30, 2002 will you receive these benefits, and **what amount** will you receive per month? Do not include your spouse's veterans education benefits.   **Months (50)** [ ]
   Amount (51) $ [ ]

Step Three: Answer all seven questions in this step.

52. Were you born before January 1, 1978? .... **Yes** ○ 1 **No** ○ 2

53. Will you be working on a master's or doctorate program (such as an MA, MBA, MD, JD, or Ph.D., etc.) during the school year 2001-2002? .... **Yes** ○ 1 **No** ○ 2

54. As of today, are you married? (Answer "Yes" if you are separated but not divorced.) .... **Yes** ○ 1 **No** ○ 2

55. Do you have children who receive more than half of their support from you? .... **Yes** ○ 1 **No** ○ 2

56. Do you have dependents (other than your children or spouse) who live with you and who receive more than half of their support from you, now and through June 30, 2002? .... **Yes** ○ 1 **No** ○ 2

57. Are you an orphan or ward of the court or were you a ward of the court until age 18? .... **Yes** ○ 1 **No** ○ 2

58. Are you a veteran of the U.S. Armed Forces? **See page 2.** .... **Yes** ○ 1 **No** ○ 2

If you (the student) answer "No" to every question in Step Three, go to Step Four.

If you answer "Yes" to any question in Step Three, skip Step Four and go to Step Five.

(If you are a graduate health profession student, your school may require you to complete Step Four even if you answered "Yes" in Step Three.)

For Help — www.ed.gov/prog_info/SFA/FAFSA

Step Four: Complete this step if you (the student) answered "No" to all questions in Step Three

59. Go to page 7 to determine who is considered a parent for this step. What is your parents' marital status as of today?

(Pick one.) Married/Remarried ○ 1   Single ○ 2   Divorced/Separated ○ 3   Widowed ○

60-63. What are your parents' Social Security Numbers and last names?
If your parent does not have a Social Security Number, enter 000-00-0000

60. FATHER'S/STEPFATHER'S SOCIAL SECURITY NUMBER
X X X – X X – X X X X

61. FATHER'S/STEPFATHER'S LAST NAME
FOR INFORMATION ONL

62. MOTHER'S/STEPMOTHER'S SOCIAL SECURITY NUMBER
X X X – X X – X X X X

63. MOTHER'S/STEPMOTHER'S LAST NAME
DO NOT SUBMIT

64. Go to page 7 to determine how many people are in your parents' household.

65. Go to page 7 to determine how many in question 64 **(exclude your parents)** will be college students between July 1, 2001 and June 30, 2002.

66. What is your parents' state of legal residence? STATE

67. Did your parents become legal residents of the state in question 66 before January 1, 1996? Yes ○ 1 No ○

68. If the answer to question 67 is "No," give the month and year legal residency began for the parent who has lived in the state the longest. MONTH YEAR /

69. What is the age of your older parent?

70. For 2000, have your parents completed their IRS income tax return or another tax return listed in **question 71**?

   a. My parents have already ○ 1 completed their return.
   b. My parents will file, but they have ○ 2 not yet completed their return.
   c. My parents are not going to file. **(Skip to question 76.)** ○

71. What income tax return did your parents file or will they file for 2000?

   a. IRS 1040 .... ○ 1
   b. IRS 1040A, 1040EZ, 1040Telefile ..... ○ 2
   c. A foreign tax return. **See Page 2.** ○ 3
   d. A tax return for Puerto Rico, Guam, American Samoa, the Virgin Islands, the Marshall Islands, the Federated States of Micronesia, or Palau. **See Page 2.** ○

72. If your parents have filed or will file a 1040, were they eligible to file a 1040A or 1040EZ? **See page 2.** Yes ○ 1 No ○ 2 Don't K

For questions 73 - 83, if the answer is zero or the question does not apply, enter 0.

73. What was your parents' adjusted gross income for 2000? Adjusted gross income is on IRS Form 1040–line 33; 1040A–line 19; 1040EZ–line 4; or Telefile–line I. $,

74. Enter the total amount of your parents' income tax for 2000. Income tax amount is on IRS Form 1040–line 51; 1040A–line 33; 1040EZ–line 10; or Telefile–line K. $,

75. Enter your parents' exemptions for 2000. Exemptions are on IRS Form 1040–line 6d or on Form 1040A–line 6d. For Form 1040EZ or Telefile, **see page 2.**

76-77. How much did your parents earn from working in 2000? Answer this question whether or not your parents filed a tax return. This information may be on their W-2 forms, or on IRS Form 1040–lines 7 + 12 + 18; 1040A–line 7; or 1040EZ–line 1. Telefilers should use their W-2's.

   Father/Stepfather (76) $,
   Mother/Stepmother (77) $,

Parent Worksheets (78-80)

78-80. Go to Page 8 and complete the columns on the right of Worksheets A, B, and C. Enter the parent totals in questions 78, 79, and 80, respectively. Even though your parents may have few of the Worksheet items, check each line carefully.

   Worksheet A (78) $,
   Worksheet B (79) $,
   Worksheet C (80) $,

81. As of today, what is the net worth of your parents' current **investments**? See page 2. $,

82. As of today, what is the net worth of your parents' current **businesses and/or investment farms**? **See page 2.** Do not include a farm that your parents live on and operate. $,

83. As of today, what is your parents' total current balance of cash, savings, and checking accounts? $,

Now go to Step Six.

Step Five: Complete this step only if you (the student) answered "Yes" to any question in Step Three.

84. Go to page 7 to determine how many people are in your (and your spouse's) household.

85. Go to page 7 to determine how many in question 84 will be college students between July 1, 2001 and June 30, 2002.

Step Six: Please tell us which schools should receive your information.

For each school (up to six), please provide the federal school code and your housing plans. Look for the federal school codes on the Internet at **www.fafsa.ed.gov**, at your college financial aid office, at your public library, or by asking your high school guidance counselor. If you cannot get the federal school code, write in the complete name, address, city, and state of the college.

86. 1ST FEDERAL SCHOOL CODE	OR	NAME OF COLLEGE / ADDRESS AND CITY — STATE — 87. HOUSING PLANS: on campus ○1 / off campus ○2 / with parent ○3
88. 2ND FEDERAL SCHOOL CODE	OR	NAME OF COLLEGE / ADDRESS AND CITY — STATE — 89. on campus ○1 / off campus ○2 / with parent ○3
90. 3RD FEDERAL SCHOOL CODE	OR	NAME OF COLLEGE / ADDRESS AND CITY — STATE — 91. on campus ○1 / off campus ○2 / with parent ○3
92. 4TH FEDERAL SCHOOL CODE	OR	NAME OF COLLEGE / ADDRESS AND CITY — STATE — 93. on campus ○1 / off campus ○2 / with parent ○3
94. 5TH FEDERAL SCHOOL CODE	OR	NAME OF COLLEGE / ADDRESS AND CITY — STATE — 95. on campus ○1 / off campus ○2 / with parent ○3
96. 6TH FEDERAL SCHOOL CODE	OR	NAME OF COLLEGE / ADDRESS AND CITY — STATE — 97. on campus ○1 / off campus ○2 / with parent ○3

Step Seven: Please read, sign, and date.

By signing this application, you agree, if asked, to provide information that will verify the accuracy of your completed form. This information may include your U.S. or state income tax forms. Also, you certify that you (1) will use federal and/or state student financial aid only to pay the cost of attending an institution of higher education, (2) are not in default on a federal student loan or have made satisfactory arrangements to repay it, (3) do not owe money back on a federal student grant or have made satisfactory arrangements to repay it, (4) will notify your school if you default on a federal student loan, and (5) understand that **the Secretary of Education has the authority to verify information reported on this application with the Internal Revenue Service.** If you purposely give false or misleading information, you may be fined $10,000, sent to prison, or both.

98. Date this form was completed.

MONTH / DAY / 2001 ○ or 2002 ○

99. Student signature   (Sign in box)

1 | **FOR INFORMATION ONLY.**

Parent signature (one parent whose information is provided in Step Four)   (Sign in box)

2 | **DO NOT SUBMIT.**

If this form was filled out by someone other than you, your spouse, or your parent(s), that person must complete this part.

Preparer's name, firm, and address

100. Preparer's Social Security Number (or 101)

101. Employer ID number (or 100)

102. Preparer's signature and date

SCHOOL USE ONLY: Federal School Code

D/O ○ 1

FAA SIGNATURE

MDE USE ONLY:
Special Handle

Notes for questions **59–83** (page 5) **Step Four:** Who is considered a parent in this step?

Read these notes to determine who is considered a parent for purposes of this form. **Answer all questions in Step Four about them**, even if you do not live with them.

If your parents are both living and married to each other, answer the questions about them.

If your parent is widowed or single, answer the questions about that parent. If your widowed parent has remarried as of today, answer the questions about that parent **and** the person whom your parent married (your stepparent).

If your parents have divorced or separated, answer the questions about the parent you lived with more during the past 12 months. (If you did not live with one parent more than the other, give answers about the parent who provided more financial support during the last 12 months, or during the most recent year that you actually received support from a parent.) If this parent has remarried as of today, answer the questions on the rest of this form about that parent **and** the person whom your parent married (your stepparent).

Notes for question **64** (page 5)

Include in your parents' household (see notes, above, for who is considered a parent):
- your parents and yourself, even if you don't live with your parents, and
- your parents' other children if (a) your parents will provide more than half of their support from July 1, 2001 through June 30, 2002 or (b) the children could answer "No" to every question in Step Three, and
- other people if they now live with your parents, your parents provide more than half of their support, and your parents will continue to provide more than half of their support from July 1, 2001 through June 30, 2002.

Notes for questions **65** (page 5) and **85** (page 6)

Always count yourself as a college student. **Do not include your parents.** Include others only if they will attend at least half time in 2001-2002 a program that leads to a college degree or certificate.

Notes for question **84** (page 6)

Include in your (and your spouse's) household.
- yourself (and your spouse, if you have one), and
- your children, if you will provide more than half of their support from July 1, 2001 through June 30, 2002, and
- other people if they now live with you, and you provide more than half of their support, and you will continue to provide more than half of their support from July 1, 2001 through June 30, 2002.

Information on the Privacy Act and use of your Social Security Number

We use the information that you provide on this form to determine if you are eligible to receive federal student financial aid and the amount that you are eligible to receive. Section 483 of the Higher Education Act of 1965, as amended, gives us the authority to ask you and your parents these questions, and to collect the Social Security Numbers of you and your parents.

State and institutional student financial aid programs may also use the information that you provide on this form to determine if you are eligible to receive state and institutional aid and the need that you have for such aid. Therefore, we will disclose the information that you provide on this form to each institution you list in questions 86–97, state agencies in your state of legal residence, and the state agencies of the states in which the colleges that you list in questions 86–97 are located.

If you are applying solely for federal aid, you must answer all of the following questions that apply to you: 1–9, 13–15, 24, 27–28, 31–32, 35, 37–40, 42–49, 52–66, 69–74, 76-85, and 98–99. If you do not answer these questions, you will not receive federal aid.

Without your consent, we may disclose information that you provide to entities under a published "routine use." Under such a routine use, we may disclose information to third parties that we have authorized to assist us in administering the above programs; to other federal agencies under computer matching programs, such as those with the Internal Revenue Service, Social Security Administration, Selective Service System, Immigration and Naturalization Service, and Veterans Administration; to your parents or spouse; and to members of Congress if you ask them to help you with student aid questions.

If the federal government, the U.S. Department of Education, or an employee of the U.S. Department of Education is involved in litigation, we may send information to the Department of Justice, or a court or adjudicative body, if the disclosure is related to financial aid and certain conditions are met. In addition, we may send your information to a foreign, federal, state, or local enforcement agency if the information that you submitted indicates a violation or potential violation of law, for which that agency has jurisdiction for investigation or prosecution. Finally, we may send information regarding a claim that is determined to be valid and overdue to a consumer reporting agency. This information includes identifiers from the record; the amount, status, and history of the claim; and the program under which the claim arose.

State Certification

By submitting this application, you are giving your state financial aid agency permission to verify any statement on this form and to obtain income information for all persons required to report income on this form.

The Paperwork Reduction Act of 1995

The Paperwork Reduction Act of 1995 says that no one is required to respond to a collection of information unless it displays a valid OMB control number, which for this form is 1845-0001. The time required to complete this form is estimated to be one hour, including time to review instructions, search data resources, gather the data needed, and complete and review the information collection. If you have comments about this estimate or suggestions for improving this form, please write to: U.S. Department of Education, Washington DC 20202-4651.

We may request additional information from you to ensure efficient application processing operations. We will collect this additional information only as needed and on a voluntary basis.

Page 7

Worksheets

Do not mail these worksheets in with your application.
Keep these worksheets; your school may ask to see them.

Worksheet A
Calendar Year 2000

For question 44 Student/Spouse		For question 78 Parent(s)
$	Earned income credit from IRS Form 1040–line 60a; 1040A–line 38a; 1040EZ–line 8a; or Telefile–line L	$
$	Additional child tax credit from IRS Form 1040–line 62 or 1040A–line 39	$
$	Welfare benefits, including Temporary Assistance for Needy Families (TANF). Don't include food stamps.	$
$	Social Security benefits received that were not taxed (such as SSI)	$
$	**Enter in question 44.** **Enter in question 78.**	$

Worksheet B
Calendar Year 2000

For question 45 Student/Spouse		For question 79 Parent(s)
$	Payments to tax-deferred pension and savings plans (paid directly or withheld from earnings), including amounts reported on the W-2 Form in Box 13, codes D, E, F, G, H, and S	$
$	IRA deductions and payments to self-employed SEP, SIMPLE, and Keogh and other qualified plans from IRS Form 1040–total of lines 23 + 29 or 1040A–line 16	$
$	Child support **received** for all children. Don't include foster care or adoption payments.	$
$	Tax exempt interest income from IRS Form 1040–line 8b or 1040A–line 8b	$
$	Foreign income exclusion from IRS Form 2555–line 43 or 2555EZ–line 18	$
$	Untaxed portions of pensions from IRS Form 1040–lines (15a minus 15b) + (16a minus 16b) or 1040A–lines (11a minus 11b) + (12a minus 12b) excluding rollovers	$
$	Credit for federal tax on special fuels from IRS Form 4136–line 9 – nonfarmers only	$
$	Housing, food, and other living allowances paid to members of the military, clergy, and others (including cash payments and cash value of benefits)	$
$	Veterans noneducation benefits such as Disability, Death Pension, or Dependency & Indemnity Compensation (DIC) and/or VA Educational Work-Study allowances	$
	Any other untaxed income or benefits not reported elsewhere on Worksheets A and B, such as worker's compensation, untaxed portions of railroad retirement benefits, Black Lung Benefits, Refugee Assistance, etc. **Don't include** student aid, Workforce Investment Act educational benefits, or benefits from flexible spending arrangements, e.g., cafeteria plans.	$
	Cash **received**, or any money paid on your behalf, not reported elsewhere on this form	XXXXXXXX
	Enter in question 45. **Enter in question 79.**	$

Worksheet C
Calendar Year 2000

For question 46 Student/Spouse		For question 80 Parent(s)
	Education credits (Hope and Lifetime Learning tax credits) from IRS Form 1040-line 46 or 1040A-line 29	$
	Child support **paid** because of divorce or separation. Do not include support for children in your (or your parents') household, as reported in question 84 (or question 64 for your parents).	$
	Taxable earnings from Federal Work-Study or other need-based work programs	$
	Student grant, scholarship, and fellowship aid, including AmeriCorps awards, that was reported to the IRS in your (or your parents') adjusted gross income	$
	Enter in question 46. **Enter in question 80.**	$

Page 8

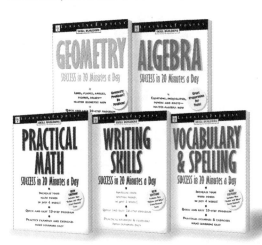
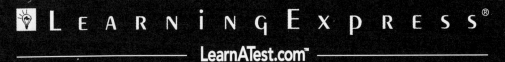

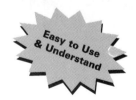
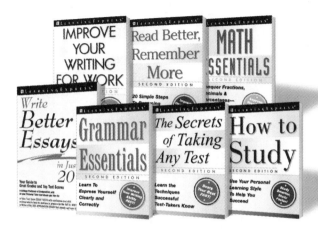
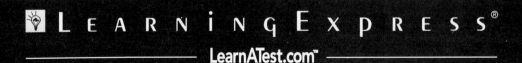